Praise from the Experts for
Macular Degeneration

"This is one of the rare books in low vision that I could not put down once I started reading. This book should be read by everyone with macular degeneration, as well as their families, friends, and doctors . . . It will be required reading for all my residents."
—RANDALL JOSE, O.D.
Director, Houston Delta Gamma Low Vision Center
Editor, *Understanding Low Vision*

"An outstanding book—not only educational but inspirational. Everyone with macular degeneration, their family members, and all eye care professionals should have a copy."
—JOEL A. KRAUT, M.D.
Medical Director, Vision Rehabilitation Service
Massachusetts Eye and Ear Infirmary
Harvard Medical School

"This book should be read, highlighted, and used as a guide by everyone who has macular degeneration, or is at risk of developing it."
—ROBERT W. MASSOF, Ph.D.
Director, Lions Vision Research and
Rehabilitation Center
Johns Hopkins University

"An excellent book! *Macular Degeneration* will be an exciting landmark in the field. I look forward to having copies available for all my patients."
—ROBERT W. CHRISTIANSEN, M.D.
Director, Low Vision Services
University of Utah

"It's about time such a valuable, comprehensive book is available for the millions who have or know someone with macular degeneration. This book will be a godsend."

—LORRAINE H. MARCHI,
Founder and Executive Director
National Association for the
Visually Handicapped (NAVH),
New York and San Francisco

"Written with remarkable understanding and sensitivity . . . This is a special book!"

—DAVID K. GIESER, M.D.
President, Wheaton Eye Clinic
Wheaton, IL

"*Macular Degeneration* is informative, down to earth, and inspiring."

—R. TRACY WILLIAMS, O.D.
Executive Director
Deicke Center for Visual Rehabilitation
Wheaton, IL

"I am so delighted that this is going to be published—it will provide a tremendous service to both patients and professionals. I look forward to providing this book to my own patients."

—DONALD C. FLETCHER, M.D.
Director, Low Vision Rehabilitation
Retina Consultants of Southwest Florida

"This is a wonderful book—it provides a wealth of clinical and personal information, enabling one to cope with macular degeneration. The authors are to be highly commended."

—GWEN K. STERNS, M.D.
Clinical Professor and Chief,
Department of Opthalmology,
Rochester General Hospital, NY

MACULAR
DEGENERATION

The Complete Guide to Saving and Maximizing Your Sight

LYLAS G. MOGK, M.D.
and MARJA MOGK

BALLANTINE BOOKS · NEW YORK

A Ballantine Book
Published by The Ballantine Publishing Group

http://www.randomhouse.com/BB/

LIBRARY OF CONGRESS CATALOGING-IN-PUBLICATION DATA
Mogk, Lylas G.
Macular degeneration : the complete guide to saving and maximizing your sight / Lylas G. Mogk, and Marja Mogk. — 1st ed.
p.   cm.
Includes bibliographical references (p. 388).
ISBN 0-345-42598-7 (trade paper : alk. paper)
1. Retinal degeneration—Popular works.
I. Mogk, Marja.   II. Title.
RE661.D3M64   1999
617.7'35—dc21   98-46041
CIP

Text design by Holly Johnson

Manufactured in the United States of America

First Edition: February 1999

10   9   8   7   6   5   4   3   2   1

For Jack and Dad
we love you

For
Charles R. Good

And for the many people with macular degeneration who are struggling to meet the challenges
of low vision with grace and humor. We will all
be seniors someday. Unless a cure for macular
degeneration is found, we, too, will experience low
vision in increasing numbers. If you have macular
degeneration you are not alone. You can still live
a fully active and engaged life for many years to
come, and you are already an inspiration to us.

CONTENTS

Contents

PART III: VISUAL REHABILITATION

PART IV: APPENDICES

Acknowledgments

We are grateful to everyone who contributed to this book and to those who generously shared their own experiences with macular degeneration so that others will not feel alone. We hope most of all that *Macular Degeneration* will be a bridge for people with ARMD to accurate information, mutual and family support, and visual rehabilitation.

We would like to acknowledge the many people who have dedicated their careers to low vision rehabilitation and education and we hope that *Macular Degeneration* will be a bridge between professionals. There are more than 1.5 million people in the United States today who need comprehensive low vision services, and so few facilities and trained professionals. There are many stretches of America where no visual rehabilitation services are available. We can never hope to meet this enormous need unless we all work together to help publicize the field, educate low vision professionals, and open the eyes of our neighbors, health care organizations, and universities to the many seniors with macular degeneration who deserve to live as fully now as they always have.

Our sincere thanks to Anne Toth Riddering, M.A., O.T.R., who designed the reading workshop program in Chapter 10, and the community and home visual rehabilitation programs in Chapters 13 and 14. She deserves credit as the coauthor of these chapters and as a wonderful colleague. We appreciate the enthusiastic support of Julian Nussbaum, M.D., Chair, Philip C. Hessburg, M.D., and colleagues at Henry Ford Eye Care Services and Grosse Pointe Ophthalmology. And we just can't say enough about the outstanding staff at the Visual Rehabilitation and Research Center of Michigan. Along with Annie, Cathy Bruce, Shannon Brafford, David Dahl, M.S., and Gary Trick, Ph.D. have made this program work. Their professional dedication and good cheer touches everyone who comes to see us. We hope we have conveyed some of their spirit in this book.

Many thanks to our family and friends: Wendy Kindred, Ed O'Malley, M.D., Lynne Mogk, Carol Gaskin, Mike and Dara Pond, Ken and Monica Payson, and Jeanne Goldberg. Wendy painted several beautiful portraits for the Charles Bonnet chapter that, to our great disappointment, could not be included. Ed drew the detailed computer illustrations of the eye for Chapter 1, Mike and Dara gave us their wedding photo, Lynne and Carol contributed the simple greens recipes, Ken and Monica spent hours in the kitchen creating the gourmet greens recipes, and Jeanne spent hours in her studio with Henry. The whole book would have been much harder to write without their support and invaluable friendship.

Acknowledgments

We are grateful to those who volunteered to talk to us about their experiences with macular degeneration. Through these conversations we both learned so much about living with low vision, and about living life itself fully and gracefully. Our best wishes always to Muriel Bleich, Geraldine Brancheau, Beatrice Brandes, John and Lucille Bukowicz, Ricky Covertt, Eloise Craig, Lillian Danluck, Dorothy Douglass, Frances Gates, Edith Goldman, Helen Konkoff, Sophie Plotzke, Genevieve Rentz, Geraldine Spaven, Steve and Gloria Sweeney, and Dorothy Wroten.

Macular Degeneration benefits greatly from the substantive suggestions and reviews by leaders in the field of low vision. The generosity with which everyone agreed to share their time and expertise was a source of great encouragement to us. We are deeply appreciative to Gary W. Abrams, M.D., Ian Bailey, O.D., Robert M. Christiansen, M.D., David Colasante, M.D., August Colenbrander, M.D., Lawrence S. Evans, M.D., Ph.D., Eleanor E. Faye, M.D., Donald C. Fletcher, M.D., David K. Gieser, M.D., Judy Gandelot, O.T., Gregory L. Goodrich, Ph.D., David R. Guyer, M.D., Clare M. Hood, R.N., M.A., Lea Hyvarinen, M.D., Randall Jose, O.D., Joel Kraut, M.D., Jeffrey Todd Liegner, M.D., Jeanine Louise, Lorraine Marchi, Robert Massof, Ph.D., L. David Ormerod, M.D., MSc., Anna Ortiz-Harder, O.T., Tomasina A. Perry, Ramona Richardson-Young, Bruce Rosenthal, O.D., Barry W. Rovner, M.D.,

Acknowledgments

David Seftell, M.D., M.B.A., Karen Seidman, M.P.A., Gwen K. Sterns, M.D., Stanley Wainapel, M.D., M.P.H., Mary Warren, M.S., O.T.R., Gale Watson, M.Ed., and R. Tracy Williams, O.D.

We would also like to thank our agent, Ruth Wreshner, and our editor, Betsy Flagler, for their faith in the project and their support; Jane Kelly, M.D., for her perceptive medical review and for her warm friendship; Bill Mogk and Helen Williams for reading the manuscript and giving great advice on organization and tone; Andrea Rogers for her reference work; Lee Lamborn for his careful editing; and, of course, Henry for her remarkable patience and companionship.

Introduction:
My Father's Story

My father and I are both night owls. When I was in high school I loved to stay up late, doing my homework in the kitchen while my father sat across the table, evaluating blueprints. A mechanical engineer by profession, my father was a consummate problem solver and a wonderfully patient math teacher. He was also an intensely visual person. He loved bird watching and photography. He built a darkroom in the basement during the 1940s and developed a portfolio that reveals his gift for design and technical detail.

In 1985, at the age of seventy-nine, my father was diagnosed with macular degeneration in one eye. For five years he was fine, until the sudden, unexpected death of my mother, his adored wife of fifty-three years. This profound loss was followed swiftly by the loss of my father's vision in his other eye from full-blown wet macular degeneration. Laser treatments could not stop the progression of the condition, and he was forced to give up driving, a significant disadvantage in the Detroit area where people and places are spread far apart. My father is a naturally cheerful soul from a long line of intrepid Hungarian-Americans, but my mother's death and his low vision were tremendous blows to him. He struggled with managing his own home alone, and struggled also with depression. I remember stopping by one afternoon, shortly after his vision had deteriorated. He was out in the yard investigating a robin's nest. "It's a shame," he said, turning to me quietly, "that Nature takes away one's sight just when we are ready to be peacefully attentive to her. I would love so much to see these birds as clearly as I once did."

Today, at ninety-three, my father has late stage macular degeneration, with 20/800 vision in one eye, and 20/500 in the other. Yet his outlook is brighter than it was several years ago. "I don't know why I outlived your mother," he told me recently, "but since I'm alive, I believe I am meant to be happy, and so I've decided to do so." He lives with my husband and me now, but he leads his life independently. He takes long walks in the neighborhood, regularly crossing intersections of every size, shops for groceries, handles his own dry cleaning, and uses the local buses. He volunteers at a low vision center, helping other seniors choose optical aids. He bowls in a league, attends monthly senior men's club lectures, dines out often, and writes his own checks. He particularly loves books on tape, and has become an avid listener. Late at night, when we are both up at the kitchen table, he'll tell me something about the cultural revolution in China or Tony Hillerman's fiction. I really think he reads more now with his ears than he used to with his eyes.

What enables him to survive, to be happy? How did he manage to meet the enormous challenge of vision loss, combined with the other colossal losses that being a senior often entails, like the loss of my mother? How did he manage to turn a larger-than-life lemon into lemonade? I found myself asking these questions often as I met more and more patients in my ophthalmology practice who also have macular degeneration. I came to realize that my father had several important advantages.

First, as an engineer, he knew something about optics and how magnifiers work, and could experiment with different models, finding the right one to maximize his sight. His problem-solving instincts and his infinite patience also helped tremendously. Just as he used to solve design impasses through rigorous inquiry and careful testing, he now figures out a way to get where he wants to go with the same approach and determination. Secondly, his sense of himself remains remarkably unshaken. He is quite straightforward about his vision loss, and doesn't hesitate to ask acquaintances to identify themselves or waiters to help with menus. He believes he is more than the sum total of his visual acuity, and he believes low vision is nothing to be embarrassed about. Finally, his daughter is an ophthalmologist, and he has access to rehabilitation services, a support group, and a full range of optical aids.

But what about the 1.5 million other Americans who have vision loss from macular degeneration and may not have these advantages? My father's experience opened my eyes to the tremendous need to provide accurate information, services, and support to people with macular degeneration and their families and friends. There may not be another medical condition in this country that is so common, that impacts daily living so profoundly, and yet is so little publicized.

In January of 1997, I opened the Visual Rehabilitation and Research Center of Michigan, part of the Henry Ford Health System, in the hopes of meeting the needs of people with macular degeneration and low vision. Our comprehensive visual rehabilitation program is called Low Vision Living. Since it began, I have been besieged with patients asking for more material. Many people are surprised to find that so many others are facing the same challenges they are, people right in their own neighborhood. Many are frustrated that there aren't better treatments, and they want to know exactly what is known about macular degeneration, and the status of current research. I have also talked to hundreds of the adult children, friends, and neighbors of people who have macular degeneration. They wonder what they can do to help, and how they can avoid getting macular degeneration, too. At sixty, with my father's light blue eyes, it's a question I ask myself. But I found little information in print that I could hand someone. So my daughter Marja and I decided to write this book to bring the Low Vision Living Program to you. It's the book I would want for my own family.

MACULAR DEGENERATION: THE COMPLETE GUIDE TO SAVING AND MAXIMIZING YOUR SIGHT IS ABOUT SAVING SIGHT IN ALL SENSES OF THE WORD

Macular Degeneration: The Complete Guide to Saving and Maximizing Your Sight is about saving sight in all senses of the word. First, it is about actually saving sight: what we can do to manage macular degeneration, and prevent it, according to what we know at this time. Part I provides a clear explanation of macular degeneration, accurate analysis of current treatments and ongoing research, and a four-point prevention program. Hopefully, *Macular Degeneration* will be a wake-up call. Hopefully it will alert the broader public to the rise of this condition as a serious public health issue, prompting the government, companies, and private foundations to increase funding for research into new modes of prevention, treatment, and visual rehabilitation.

This book is also about the sight you will

always keep, even if you have advanced macular degeneration. Macular degeneration does not blind. It leaves peripheral vision intact, and this remaining vision is a saving grace. You can learn to maximize your remaining sight through optical aids and rehabilitation, and it will take you a long way on the road to maintaining a lifestyle you enjoy. For this purpose, Part III provides a complete home visual rehabilitation program. The appendices also list resources for finding professional visual rehabilitation programs in your area and low vision products.

Finally, the phrase *saving sight* raises the question of what it means, exactly, to save sight or what it means to provide medical care for vision. Oliver Sacks tells the true story of a man who, born blind, lived his whole life seeing with his hands. As a middle-aged adult, his doctors restored his sight surgically. But the cure left him profoundly depressed. He found it tremendously difficult to adjust to a world full of bombarding images, and felt adrift without his familiar identity as a blind person. Sacks's story points to the heart of a critical weakness in medicine that is no less evident in ophthalmology than in any other specialty: doctors are typically trained to treat a particular part of the body, but not the whole person. We are so focused on eyes that we rarely take into consideration the context in which people live and how they see their own lives.

But individuals are not all eyeball, and

macular degeneration doesn't happen in a vacuum. It's part and parcel of a whole life lived by a whole person. *Macular Degeneration: The Complete Guide* is about the saving power of insight. It's about the power of doctors and therapists understanding the context and consequences of low vision. It's about the power of family and friends understanding the whole experience of low vision. And it's about people with macular degeneration seeing themselves as so much more than a pair of eyes. Part II addresses the experience of macular degeneration, providing a framework for coping with low vision, and sharing the thoughts and words of some of the people with macular degeneration whom we have had the honor to know.

PART I:

Understanding ARMD

CHAPTER I

What is ARMD?
A Portrait

Macular degeneration is one of the
biggest secrets in the world.
> —Emil F. Hubka, Jr.
> ARMD patient

This has become a true epidemic of
our time.
> —Jerry Chader, Ph.D.
> Chief Scientific Officer
> The Foundation Fighting Blindness

"I thought I needed new glasses," Zelda Grant
remembers. "I was shocked to discover that I have
age-related macular degeneration. 'Macular what?'
I said to my doctor. I had never heard of it before,
and I could hardly believe that some disease I had
never heard of was stealing my eyesight." Alarm-
ingly, Zelda's experience is very common. Age-
Related Macular Degeneration, or ARMD, is the
leading cause of adult vision loss in the United
States. It affects more people than all of the better
known eye diseases combined: glaucoma, cataracts,

and diabetic retinopathy. According to the respected Beaver Dam Eye Study—the most comprehensive attempt to estimate the demographics of macular degeneration in the United States—18 percent of seniors aged sixty-five to seventy-four and nearly 30 percent of seniors over seventy-five show early evidence of the condition. One out of every twenty-five Americans over sixty-five, or 1,367,000 people, suffers significant vision loss from advanced macular degeneration. Clearly, if you have ARMD you are not alone.

What is Age-Related Macular Degeneration?

Macular degeneration dismantles central vision painlessly and silently, leaving peripheral vision intact. As a result, people with advanced macular degeneration do not feel any change in their eyes, and they do not appear any different to their friends and family, but their experience of the world and of their own capacities changes radically. Because macular degeneration leaves peripheral vision intact, people with ARMD can see whatever rests at the edges of their vision, but cannot see clearly whatever they look at directly. They find it difficult to recognize their grandchildren's photographs, for example, but can describe the check pattern of a black and white tile floor. They cannot read a bus sign, but can see a leaf on the sidewalk out of the corners of their eyes. This combination of visual ability and vision loss is enormously frustrating, not the least because it takes away what we most want to see, leaving visible what appears to be irrelevant. As Carolyn See, an English professor, remarks dryly in her candid memoir of living with macular degeneration, "It begins in the center of your vision and after a while you can't read or drive or recognize your relatives. They say you'll always be able to pick up a thread on the carpet. But even with full vision, picking up threads on the carpet wasn't high on my list of activities."

Why Has Macular Degeneration Been a Big Secret?

Macular degeneration is coming out of the closet. Three years ago, patients came to appointments asking me to check their eyes for signs of glaucoma. Today they arrive asking about macular degeneration. But macular degeneration has been a leading cause of vision loss in seniors for decades. Why did it take us until the late 1990s to talk about it? No one is quite sure.

The first explanation may lie in the physiology of ARMD. Even though macular degeneration was first named by a German scientist in 1885, the technology used to understand it in detail was not developed until the 1960s. Unlike cataracts, which can easily be seen, or glaucoma, which can easily be measured, macular degeneration is more difficult to analyze and to treat. Ophthalmologists have tended to focus their energies on developing fine new surgeries that have helped improve the sight of hundreds of thousands of people with many different eye conditions. But macular degeneration never looked like a condition that would respond readily to surgery, so it wound up a bit lower on the research priority list.

A second explanation of why ARMD has not been talked about may lie in the category of people affected by it: seniors. Until about ten years ago, ARMD was called senile macular degeneration, which may be another clue to its anonymity. Although *senile* is a word we commonly associate with declining mental health, *senile macular degeneration* simply means macular degeneration in older people. But no matter how you define it, senile still connotes decline, and for much of this century declining vision was simply accepted as the result of "just growing old." But seniors like Zelda and Carolyn are now living longer and in better health than their parents and grandparents. Healthy longevity is on the rise: a sixty-five-year-old may have twenty to forty more years of reading, entertaining, traveling, and sports ahead of her; she may not even feel ready to retire. Seniors today are also less willing to accept adversity from aging as quietly as their parents and grandparents did. Zelda and her peers want to know, justifiably, why there is so little attention paid to macular degeneration, why their insurance companies don't cover visual aids or therapy for low vision, and when a cure will be developed. Vision loss is no longer an expected part of just growing old, nor should it be.

Macular Degeneration Gains Attention

Macular degeneration has become a major health issue, and more and more physicians, pharmaceutical companies, and laboratories are searching for cures and for a clearer understanding of what causes ARMD. But even with this new attention, the total amount of research dollars devoted to ARMD is still small considering that it is the biggest cause of irreversible vision loss in the country: more than cataracts, glaucoma, and diabetic retinopathy combined. The National Eye Institute (NEI), a division of the National Institutes of Health, has ranked ARMD its number one priority, but for the magnitude of the problem a relatively small percentage of the national health budget is devoted specifically to ARMD research. Unless we speak up, this situation is unlikely to change, and prevention and cure will be that many more years away.

Many seniors depend on the American Association of Retired Persons (AARP) to lobby Washington on their behalf, but the AARP follows a policy of not addressing any one disease. That means there is no major voice in Washington telling Congress that macular degeneration research is important to Americans. Write your representatives in Congress and ask them to support the NEI and promote additional funding for macular degeneration research. Fortunately, ARMD has been in the news enough that they should understand the urgency of your request.

Newsweek, *Time*, *Prevention*, *US News and World Report*, *The New York Times*, and CNN have all reported on new studies since early 1996. News reports, however, are not always entirely complete. While celebrating and encouraging scientific breakthroughs, the media have a tendency to trumpet results prematurely. Experimental treatments and special curative diets are sometimes presented as if their success has already been confirmed. The hopes of many combined with the relative lack of public information on the topic (at least until 1999) give these news reports great weight. Patients often call to ask about new cures and requesting treatments that haven't really been proven effective or safe. The truth is that macular degeneration is complicated; there is no easy answer. Chapter 2, "ARMD Treatments and Medical Research," and Chapter 3, "Genes and Greens: The Causes and Prevention of ARMD," accurately explain the latest information on research, treatment, and prevention. It is important to understand what we really do and do not know, and it's also important to keep faith in the future since it will hold new solutions.

Macular Degeneration Isn't Just About Your Eyes

Unfortunately, few authorities recognize that ARMD affects more than a person's eyes. Most people say they'd rather lose a limb than an eye, and national surveys tend to place vision loss among the most feared afflictions, along with cancer. Why? Because eyesight affects every aspect of life: mobility, physical activity, communication, appearance, perception, self-esteem, and psychological health. Macular degeneration is not just about how much you can or cannot see. It's about your whole life: how you cope with change, your view of the future, and your capacity to enjoy the present. And macular degeneration is tailor-made to push every button we have. It can raise feelings of grief, helplessness, depression, fear, anxiety, and anger. This book seeks to address these experiences in Part II, but first we have to define the condition itself. As Zelda put it, "macular what?" What is macular degeneration anyway?

AGE-RELATED MACULAR DEGENERATION EXPLAINED

Our Eyes Are Like Little Cameras

You have probably heard this analogy before: our eyes are like little cameras.

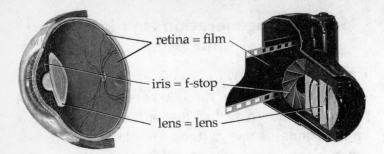

retina = film

iris = f-stop

lens = lens

The human eye is like a camera. While the film is simply a strip in the back of the camera, the retina lines the entire inside of the eyeball.

Just as light enters the camera through the shutter, is focused by the lens, and falls on the film, so light enters our eye through the pupil, is focused by the lens, and falls on the retina at the back of our eye. The retina is like camera film. Its thin tissue forms the inner lining of the eye, picking up light and converting it into nerve signals. The retina sends those signals through the optic nerve to the brain, which "develops" them into the images we actually see, just as film is developed into photographs.

The Macula: Center of the Retina

The retina has two types of photoreceptor cells that convert light into electrical messages for the optic nerve to transmit: rod cells and cone cells, so named for their shapes. There are many more rods than cones throughout the retina, especially at the edges, where rods outnumber cones twenty to one. Rod cells are responsible for peripheral vision and light-and-dark contrast perception. They essentially provide us with background information, but they cannot transmit crisp pictures. We use the rods of our peripheral vision to catch a glimpse of something. They tell us that a car is coming from the far left or right, but in order to see the car clearly or describe it, we instinctively turn to look at it directly. As soon as we turn, however, we are no longer primarily

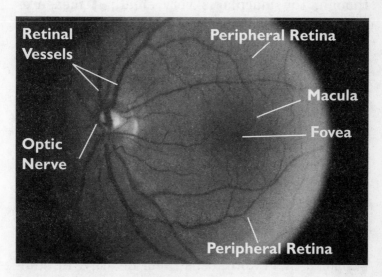

Photograph of the inside of a normal eye. This is what doctors see when they look into your eye.

using our rod cells to see, but our cone cells. Cones are concentrated in the center of the retina—called the macula—and are responsible for central vision, color perception, and sharp images (acute vision). The capacity of cones to distinguish detail is one hundred times greater than rods. We need them to tell the difference between forest green and black, and to see precise detail, like the features of a face, the lace pattern on a table cloth, or the letters on this page. The macula is therefore both the geographic center of the retina, and the focal center of our vision. The fovea is the very center of the macula. It is also the only area of the retina that has only cone cells. For all its power, though, the macula is very small; it measures about a quarter inch in diameter and is tissue-paper thin. But the macula is truly a mouse that roars. This tiny area is responsible for so much of what we see.

Macular Degeneration: The Key Players

In macular degeneration, rod and cone cells of the macula begin to die, reducing the number of cells able to transmit visual signals to the brain. Macular degeneration, however, is not a condition of these cells alone, but of the underlying tissue that supports them and keeps them healthy. In addition to the rods and cones, there are three more key players in macular degeneration: the retinal pigment epithelium (RPE), Bruch's membrane, and the choroid. In that order, each is a layer of tissue that lies beneath the retina, like layers of a club sandwich or, more accurately, stations on a delivery line. Taken together, they form a kind of conveyor belt for nutrition and waste management, constantly supplying the macula with oxygen-laden macula meals and whisking away waste. The large blood vessels of the choroid truck materials in and out through the blood stream. Bruch's membrane acts as a security gate between these blood vessels and the delicate RPE, and the RPE delivers oxygen and receives waste directly from the rod and cone cells in the macula.

Normally, the system works very efficiently. But if there's a jam somewhere, the oxygen meal

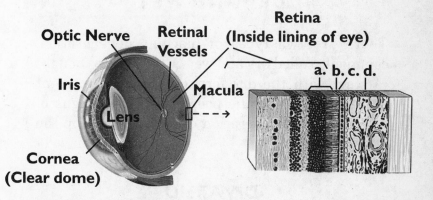

Eye showing cross section of the "conveyor belt." a: cones and rods, b: Retinal Pigment Epithelium (RPE), c: Bruch's Membrane, d: Choroid

shipments and the waste removals back up, and eventually the pick-up and drop-off stations shut down. The choroid, Bruch's membrane, and the RPE become disabled and can no longer do their jobs. When they fail, the rod and cone cells lack the massive amounts of oxygen they need to stay alive and have no way to clear away the waste products they produce by metabolizing oxygen. Dying of oxygen deprivation and clogged with refuse, rods and cones become unable to send signals through the optic nerve to the brain—they are no longer able to see. This is what happens with macular degeneration.

TWO TYPES OF ARMD: DRY AND WET

There are two types of macular degeneration, commonly called dry and wet. All cases are thought to start with the dry form. Between 10 percent and 15 percent of the people who show signs of dry macular degeneration eventually develop the wet form.

Dry ARMD

Although there is only one kind of dry ARMD, you may hear it called "atrophic," "geographic atrophy," or "nonexudative" macular degeneration. Atrophic or atrophy refers to a declining, weakening, or wasting away. We often use the word to talk about muscles that haven't been used in a great while and lose their strength as a result. We can exercise our muscles and regain strength but, unlike our muscles, atrophy in our macula isn't currently reversible. This is because the macula atrophies from a lack of oxygen, not a lack of use. And as we know, any part of our body that suffers a prolonged lack of oxygen usually sustains permanent damage. Geographic atrophy of the macula means atrophy concentrated in one contiguous area of the macula. Nonexudative means not exuding, or not discharging, meaning that there is no blood leakage in the macula contributing to the malfunctioning of the conveyor belt system.

Hard and Soft Drusen

Dry ARMD is usually signaled by the presence in the macula of small pale spots called *drusen*. There are two types of drusen: less harmful hard drusen and more ominous soft drusen. Hard drusen are small, round, sharply defined light yellow deposits of lipid (a fatty compound) and calcium that accumulate on Bruch's membrane. They are quite common with age, appearing in most older eyes like age spots appear on skin, and are not necessarily thought to indicate macular degeneration. Soft drusen can be nearly twice the size of hard drusen, with indistinct margins and varying sizes and shapes. While soft drusen can be seen in older eyes that don't develop full-blown ARMD, they have been considered an early indicator of the condition, perhaps because they are the first feature of ARMD that we can detect in an affected eye. Recently, however, researchers have suggested that by the time we can see soft drusen in an eye, macular degeneration may already be advanced.

Soft drusen are thought to plug up the conveyor belt system in dry macular degeneration. Some researchers also believe that soft drusen are responsible for wet macular degeneration because they may weaken Bruch's membrane or because they may trigger the proliferation of abnormal blood vessels. Other researchers disagree, arguing that soft drusen occur because Bruch's membrane has already been weakened for some other reason. In any case, soft drusen signal to us that the conveyor belt support system for the macula is malfunctioning and Bruch's membrane is weak, which may allow abnormal blood vessels from the choroid to creep through. Your ophthalmologist can see hard and soft drusen in your eyes during a standard eye exam, with no special testing. Your retina is transparent, although it appears red-orange because the underlying RPE gives it color. The light yellow color of the drusen shows up against this red-orange glow.

Like soft drusen, focal hyperpigmentation is another signal of possible early macular degeneration that your ophthalmologist can see. Focal hyperpigmentation means the appearance of dark-ish irregular specks in the macula. They are caused by pigment cells that clump up over time, although we aren't sure exactly why they do. When our eyes are young, healthy, and working well, they have a kind of robust color, like a rosy apple. The RPE glows bright red-orange, and the fovea, the center part of the macula, has a pretty gold glow. But when our eyes become much older or unhealthy, they appear sallow. Light yellow drusen tone down the bright red-orange of the RPE, and darkish pigment specks mark the gold of the fovea. Since age-related macular degeneration is a condition of deterioration, these age spots, like drusen, are often indicators of oncoming macular degeneration.

Wet ARMD

Wet ARMD is called "wet" because it is characterized by abnormal, leaky blood vessels that grow underneath the retina in the choroid. You may also hear wet ARMD called "subretinal net," "subretinal neovascularization" (SRNV), or "choroidal neovascularization" (CNV). Subretinal means "underneath the retina" or "underneath the RPE," and neovascularization simply means "new vessels." Wet ARMD may also be referred to as exudative degeneration. Exudative means "seeping" or "bleeding," referring to these abnormal blood vessels. We don't know why these abnormal blood

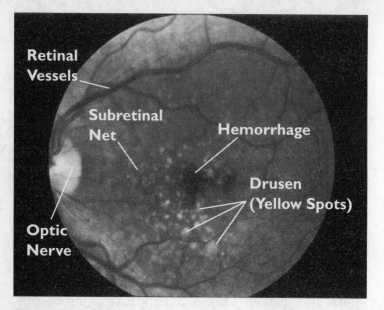

Photograph of the inside of an eye with wet ARMD, showing drusen, hemorrhage and subretinal net.

vessels grow. They grow from the choroid through Bruch's membrane, which is not supposed to allow such a thing, and collect under the RPE like tree roots under a sidewalk. These vessels are weak and tend to leak fluid and blood, which seeps through the surrounding tissue, flooding the cone cells of the macula and either suffocating them or triggering changes that result in their death. Very late stage wet macular degeneration is sometimes called disciform degeneration. Although this refers to the disc-shaped scars that result after bleeding occurs, disciform degeneration is generally used to simply refer to extensive or late stage degeneration.

If these leaky vessels exert enough pressure under the RPE, they may rip it away from Bruch's membrane, creating a sort of blister between the two layers that permanently destroys the conveyor belt system in that particular area. This condition is called a serous pigment epithelial detachment, or PED. A PED is sometimes referred to in patient information pamphlets as a third type of macular degeneration, but it is a possible development in wet macular degeneration.

Your ophthalmologist may be able to detect the presence of abnormal blood vessels in your eye because they sometimes give the affected area of your retina a muted gray-green color. But to define the precise size and shape of these vessels, a fluorescein angiogram is necessary. This is a photograph of your eye taken with a special camera that can detect dye in the blood vessels underneath your retina. Having a fluorescein angiogram involves having dye injected into your arm. This dye travels throughout your blood stream, making all of your blood, including the blood in those abnormal vessels, glow for the camera. Chapter 2 provides a more detailed explanation of fluorescein angiograms and treatments for macular degeneration.

ARMD DOES NOT AFFECT PERIPHERAL VISION

Macular degeneration is by definition a condition affecting only the macula—*not* the entire retina. It is a failure of the conveyor belt system that exclusively supports the macula, which has a very different support system from the rest of the retina. This is because the macula is the only area of the retina with a high concentration of cone cells, and cones turn out to be very high maintenance. They demand enormous quantities of oxygen, and produce enormous quantities of oxygenated waste. In fact, the macula has the highest blood flow of any area in the body. Rod cells, on the other hand, consume much less oxygen, so they don't require the same level of support. As a result, rods outside the macula have their own support system. And it doesn't clog up, partly because rods consume less oxygen and produce less waste, and partly because the rods outside the macula are distributed over a much larger area, so there is more support tissue available for each cell. It might help to think of the macula as a busy little island in the middle of a big, calm retina rod-lake: the macula has its own soil, its own root system, and its own drama of health and survival.

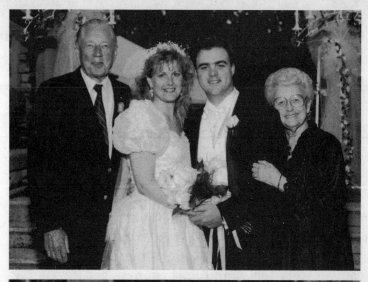

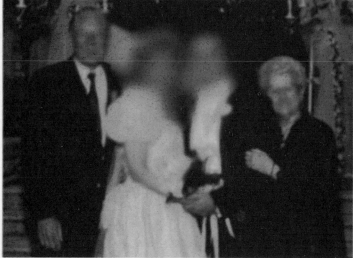

Macular degeneration damages or destroys central vision, but doesn't affect the rest of the visual field. When the center is gone, the best remaining vision is at the edges of the lost central field. This example shows mild ARMD.

PATTERNS OF ARMD PROGRESSION

Macular degeneration often catches people off guard. Not only does the disease progress painlessly and silently, but our eyes are designed to compensate for one another. If one eye's vision deteriorates gradually enough, the brain simply pays attention to the visual signals of the other eye, allowing us to maximize our vision and avoid the distractions of minor impairments. Buddy Burmester, for example, began to notice that it was more difficult to read the morning paper in his kitchen, so he turned on an extra light or sat in the sun on the deck, without really noticing his own adjustment. It wasn't until street signs became difficult to see at dusk that he thought he might need new glasses. Like Zelda, he was utterly shocked to discover that his eyesight in his right eye was 20/200, at the level of legal blindness, while his left eye was holding its own at 20/50. Buddy's experience is very common.

Visual Indications of ARMD

If you see an ophthalmologist or optometrist who checks your retinas at least every two years, he or she will likely detect early macular degeneration before you experience any significant vision loss. If you do not see an ophthalmologist or optometrist regularly, you will not be able to tell whether or not you have early macular degeneration. Like Buddy, you may not notice anything at all until you experience significant vision loss, especially if your degeneration is advanced in only one eye. You can use the Amsler Grid in Chapter 2 to test your own vision at home, but I recommend checkups with an ophthalmologist or optometrist every two years, not only for macular degeneration but also for glaucoma and for the general health of your eyes. If you do experience vision loss from macular degeneration, you are most likely to notice difficulty reading, seeing small details, pouring champagne or coffee (especially if whatever you are pouring is the same shade as your glass or cup), and distinguishing between similiar colors and subtle shades. You may also notice that you need more light to do what you used to be able to do with less light but that you are more sensitive to glare.

Your Risk of Vision Loss from Macular Degeneration

If you have a few soft drusen, which is usually considered a sign of early onset ARMD, you may never develop late stage macular degeneration and significant vision loss. The risk, however, increases with age and with other factors, like eye color, family background, a history of smoking, and nutrition. There are no reliable risk statistics for dry ARMD, which means that we cannot really predict how fast your dry macular degeneration may progress, whether you will get it in both eyes, or what amount of vision you may lose. We can use the Beaver Dam Eye Study statistics, which combine the rates of wet and dry macular degeneration, to give you a ballpark risk figure. What remains clear is that everyone's risk of macular degeneration increases with age. If you are fifty-five, for example, your chance of having early signs of macular degeneration is 13.8 percent and your chance of having full-blown macular degeneration (either wet or dry) is about .6 percent. By the time you are over seventy-five, however, those figures jump to 29.7 percent and 7.1 percent, respectively.

What Are the Risks of Developing Wet ARMD in a Second Eye?

Researchers have focused most of their efforts on wet macular degeneration since wet macular degeneration may respond to laser and causes vision loss more quickly and extensively than the dry form. For wet macular degeneration, we have more accurate risk predictions from the Macular Photocoagulation Study. This study addressed a number of specific questions, including: "What are the chances of developing wet macular degeneration in your second eye if you already have it in one eye?" The answer turns out to be: "It depends." It depends upon whether or not you have one or more of four risk factors. They are:

1. Five or more drusen in your second eye
2. More than one druse larger than .064 millimeters
3. Focal hyperpigmentation
4. High blood pressure

Your risk of developing wet macular degeneration in your second eye within five years of the first eye is as follows, according to the study:

With	no risk factors	= 7 percent
With	1 risk factor	= 25 percent
With	2 risk factors	= 44 percent
With	3 risk factors	= 53 percent
With	4 risk factors	= 87 percent

Now, there's a great deal that these figures don't tell us: how much vision you may lose in either eye, or what your chances of developing wet macular degeneration in the first eye are to start with. What they do tell us is that macular degeneration and vision loss vary greatly from one person to another. We know that you can develop macular degeneration before you experience any significant vision loss from the condition. And, as we know from Buddy Burmester's experience, you can experience significant vision loss before you realize that you have developed macular degeneration. How fast you may experience vision loss and how much vision you will lose depends, but upon what it depends is not yet clear.

As a result, people's experiences of ARMD vary greatly. Buddy Burmester, who has dry ARMD, lost vision in both eyes within four years from the time of his diagnosis. He still reads with the help of a closed circuit television, but he doesn't drive. Zelda Grant turned out to have fast progressing wet ARMD and experienced pronounced vision loss in less than six months. But their neighbor, Dolores Lopez, was diagnosed with dry ARMD in one eye nearly eight years ago, and she's still using the other eye to drive and read. Why is Dolores's macular degeneration progressing so much more slowly than Buddy's? Why didn't she develop wet macular degeneration like Zelda did? We just aren't sure. Fortunately, new studies, and even whole new centers devoted to macular degeneration research and treatment, are appearing even as you read this book. With increased attention to the condition and more research money, we will have better answers to these questions. We may also find effective ways to slow the progress of ARMD or prevent it altogether.

LATE STAGE ARMD

Given that we can't predict how macular degeneration may affect any particular person, what is the worst case scenario? Now that Buddy's and Zelda's macular degeneration has affected both of their eyes, how much vision can they expect to lose in the long run? How bad does it get? What exactly does "developing vision loss" mean anyway? The phrase sounds like a polite euphemism, largely because we have an impoverished vocabulary for talking about visual impairment. Until very recently, our options were to talk about having normal vision or being blind, with the confusing third term "legal blindness" in the mix.

Total Blindness

The good news is that Buddy and Zelda will not become totally blind from macular degeneration, and neither will anyone else. If you have ARMD and no other eye condition you will always have your peripheral vision. This sight is yours to keep, a saving grace that will enable you to always maintain a level of independence and to enjoy activities that require some vision. This is a fact, but it's a fact that many people with vision loss often doubt. When my daughter set out to interview several of my patients for this book, she discovered that at least 50 percent questioned my enthusiastic assurances that they weren't going totally blind.

At first I thought that maybe I hadn't communicated my assurances strongly enough. Then I realized that the very nature of macular degeneration fosters this doubt. As I've admitted, we don't know a great deal about its causes. And if physicians don't know exactly what causes the development of soft drusen or the proliferation of abnormal blood vessels in the macula, then how can they guarantee that total blindness from macular degeneration isn't a possibility? The answer is that this guarantee is built into the anatomy of your eye. As I explain in greater detail in the section above entitled "ARMD Does Not Affect Peripheral Vision," macular degeneration by definition is specifically a degeneration of the macula—*not* the entire retina. The rod cells that provide your peripheral vision and are located outside the macula remain unaffected by macular degeneration.

The Fear of Total Blindness

The fear of total blindness many people express may stem from the experience of having macular degeneration itself. Since ARMD is a degenerative condition, it subjects those who have it to the frustrating process of watching their eyesight slip away. Each degree of vision loss may feel like a threat to daily life, creating a timed progression that measures one year against the previous one, one day against the next. Last year I could read the newspaper, this year I cannot. Tomorrow the salt shaker will disappear. It's enough to drive even the most stalwart personality nuts. It is also enough to give the very real impression that there is no end, that the deterioration will continue endlessly until there is nothing left to lose. This impression becomes stronger as the condition progresses because the majority of remaining vision is peripheral, and peripheral vision is not very precise. As a result, it becomes more difficult to tell whether or not one's vision is as good today as it was yesterday. The remaining peripheral vision also feels very precarious, like the last lone cowboy standing on an exposed bluff. And it feels inadequate compared with fully functioning central vision.

"How much more vision can I lose and still see?" This is the question that many patients would like to throw at their doctors' assurances that they are not at risk of total blindness. What, in other words, is the practical difference between what you are calling total blindness and what I'm seeing, or more precisely, what I'm not seeing? The practical difference is enormous, especially if you work to enhance your remaining eyesight through visual rehabilitation. Vision that is 20/400, while not close to 20/20, is a great deal more sight than we commonly call blindness. My 93-year-old father has 20/500 vision in his best eye from macular degeneration. He bowls in a league, writes his own checks, and dines out regularly. He recently took a bus up to the frame shop, had his favorite photograph enlarged, gave instructions for cropping it, and selected a matching silver frame. And then he walked home. That's a lot more than he could do if he truly couldn't see anything at all.

OUR VOCABULARY OF VISION

We often think of 20/20 vision as perfect sight. We say "hindsight is 20/20" or we name a truth-finding television program *20/20*. The truth is that 20/20 vision is not perfect vision but *standard vision*, or the lowest amount of vision that is considered normal (many people have better than 20/20 vision). The first 20 represents you standing twenty feet away from an object. The second figure, in this case also a 20, represents how far away from the object a person with standard normal eyes could stand and still see it in the same amount of detail as you do. In other words, if your vision is 20/60, it means that what you can see from a distance of 20 feet, the average person with normal eyes can see from a distance of 60 feet. We can take Buddy Burmester as an example. When he discovered that the vision in his right eye was measuring 20/200, it meant that he could see at 20 feet away what his wife or daughter could see in the same detail at 200 feet away.

This figure, however, doesn't give a complete picture of the quality of Buddy's vision or of our own. There are a whole host of other variables that go into measuring visual acuity that the figures 20/60 or 20/200 don't represent. For example, 20/60 doesn't measure visual ability in varying weather or lighting conditions, and it doesn't measure color perception or contrast sensitivity. The only other measure that has gained as widespread a use as the 20/20 measure is the field measure. The average normal eye has a visual field of roughly 170 degrees, or a little less than a half circle. This means that when you look straight ahead and stretch out your arms to either side, you can see from the tip of one hand to the tip of the other out of the corners of your eyes. This is the rod cell peripheral vision that people with macular degeneration keep.

Vision Exists on a Continuum

Using the 20/20 measure as our sole vocabulary for vision is misleading because it suggests to us that seeing is an all-or-nothing proposition, rather than a process. We talk about whether we have 20/20 vision or not. We measure our sight based on a number we get from the optometrist's or ophthalmologist's office rather than on what we can accomplish with our eyes. We fall into thinking that there are two categories of people in the world: those who can see and those who can't, or the normal and the blind. But vision exists on a continuum, like hearing or feeling pain. Whenever we experience pain we are aware of its quality and intensity. Doctors often ask, "On a scale of one to ten, how much back pain do you feel?" We think of hearing on a relative scale, too. Music that one person experiences as too loud, another may experience as not loud enough. When someone says they are "hard of hearing" we accept that they have some amount of hearing loss, but we aren't sure how much—it depends upon the individual. This variation is true of vision, too.

Lorraine Marchi, a pioneer advocate in the field of low vision and the founder of The National Association for the Visually Handicapped (NAVH), coined the term *hard of seeing* as a more accurate description for most types of vision loss than the word *blind* connotes. Many blind people perceive some light, and may recognize light sources, or even see some hand motion. People with low vision see much more than hand motion, but less than about 20/60. That's a very big range. We need to get used to thinking about *low vision*, rather than *perfect vision* versus *blindness*. Low vision includes a wide range of visual ability that is less than 20/20 but more than blind. Simply, as Mrs. Marchi says, it's "hard of seeing."

Low Vision

Using *low vision* avoids the limitations of other terms like *20/20*, *blind*, or *legally blind*. And the term approximates what is actually going on, which is the presence of vision with impairment. It's a term we can use to talk about the varieties of vision that people experience, rather than continually struggling with the twin poles of perfect vision and total blindness. Because the term is new, and covers such a wide range of visual abilities, low vision is defined slightly differently by various health, government, and private organizations. Insurance reimbursement policies and state regulations differ quite a bit. For example, many states require 20/40 vision or better for an unrestricted driver's license, while others allow people with vision of 20/100 to drive. The National Eye Institute (NEI) eschews a particular acuity measurement for low vision, recommending instead that low vision be defined in terms of ability. We ought to be asking, in other words, whether or not someone can read a newspaper, or a canned goods label, or recognize a friend on the street when we seek to assess low vision.

Legal Blindness

Legal blindness does not mean total blindness. The term *legal blindness* appeared during the Great Depression. It was originally called *economic blindness* and was an arbitrary measure set by the government to determine which citizens would find it difficult to get employment as a result of impaired vision. Special economic relief programs were initiated for the people who qualified. The government designation of legally blind still stands today, and if you qualify you are entitled to a number of helpful programs and benefits detailed in Appendix II. Legal blindness is defined as having 20/200 sight in your best eye with correction, or a visual field of 20 degrees or less. This means that with glasses or contacts you can see at 20 feet with your best eye what a normal eye sees at 200 feet, or that your sight encompasses an area that is 20 degrees wide rather than 170 degrees. More than 85 percent of the people who qualify as legally blind have some functional vision; only 15 percent are completely blind. As with the 20/20 measure itself, legal blindness is an arbitrary point selected for public policy purposes. It's a great idea, but it doesn't give us details about the people who fall into the category of legally blind, many of whom have jobs that require sight. There are many people who are legally blind who absolutely do not consider themselves blind.

GLAUCOMA, CATARACTS, AND MACULAR DEGENERATION

Finally, people often ask me if glaucoma, cataracts, or diabetic retinopathy aggravate macular degeneration, or if macular degeneration aggravates any of them. The answer is no. Glaucoma, cataracts, and diabetic retinopathy are unrelated to macular degeneration. ARMD is not directly related to any other disease or eye condition to our knowledge. There is some new evidence that cataract *surgery* may affect macular degeneration, although these findings have not been widely confirmed. Chapter 2 discusses this possible relationship in greater detail. To understand why glaucoma, cataracts, and macular degeneration are unrelated, it may help to return to our original picture of the eye and clarify how each of these conditions causes vision loss.

Cataracts are opacities of the lens at the front of the eye. They prevent images and light from entering the eye, somewhat the way sheer curtains block the view through a window. Cataracts can usually be surgically removed and replaced by new lenses.

Glaucoma is a condition of high pressure inside your eye that damages your optic nerve. Your eye is

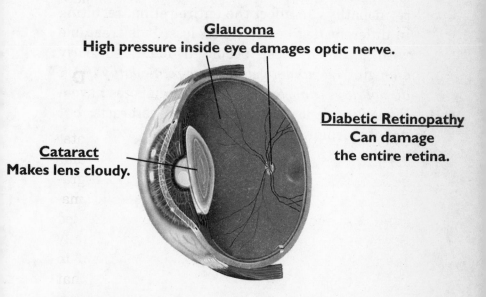

Glaucoma
High pressure inside eye damages optic nerve.

Diabetic Retinopathy
Can damage
the entire retina.

Cataract
Makes lens cloudy.

Glaucoma, cataracts and diabetic retinopathy affect the eye differently from **ARMD**. They are not related conditions.

a closed, fluid-filled system. If too much fluid accumulates, pressure inside the eye rises, pushing on the optic nerve and gradually damaging its delicate fibers. If detected early, glaucoma is easily treatable in most people with prescription eye drops, laser, or surgery. If untreated or uncontrolled, glaucoma can cause peripheral vision loss and eventually complete blindness.

Diabetic retinopathy is a condition caused by diabetes in which the retina may be swollen and abnormal blood vessels may develop on the surface of the retina. These vessels can bleed or constrict and cause retinal detachment. Diabetic retinopathy can affect the entire retina, resulting in different degrees of vision loss. It is treatable with laser in most people if identified early enough. *You cannot get diabetic retinopathy if you do not have diabetes.* People with diabetes have a higher incidence of glaucoma and cataracts, but not of macular degeneration.

CHAPTER 2

ARMD Treatments and Medical Research

Therapy for macular degeneration is
at an exciting frontier.
—<u>The Ophthalmology Times</u>
August 1995

Macular Degeneration is the number
one priority of the National Eye
Institute.
—Carl Kupfer, M.D.
Director, NEI
June 1998

Currently, laser photocoagulation is the only
medical treatment proven to be useful for ARMD,
but it can only treat wet macular degeneration. It
delays additional vision loss in 70 percent of the
people who receive treatment (7 percent of all
macular degeneration patients). There is no treatment for dry macular degeneration as yet. This is
an abysmal state of affairs for everyone. People
with ARMD want to know why there isn't any
reliable treatment. Researchers are conscientiously

searching for solutions. The media often trumpets preliminary advances in technology as available cures, causing confusion for the public. And doctors sometimes feel useless. If you've spent your whole life believing that you can help someone with your surgical and medical skills, meeting macular degeneration means that you've met your match, at least for now. As one of my colleagues confessed recently, "We feel absolutely horrible that we can't offer anything that will really cure macular degeneration. And then we have to tell someone the bad news. It's an awful feeling. One of the saddest meetings I ever attended was at a national ophthalmology meeting about four years ago. Every retinal specialist I can think of was there. They stood together on stage, hung their heads, and said, 'We don't have anything really effective to offer.' "

But laser *has* saved sight for many people. So what is laser? Is it for you? And why does medical progress on ARMD seem so slow? Why are there so many reports of treatments in the media but only laser is available? And what answers can we expect in the future? These are all questions my patients have asked many times, and we aim to answer them in this chapter.

As *The Ophthalmology Times* pointed out, this is an exciting time in the field of macular degeneration. More and more researchers are dedicating their careers to finding a cure for macular degeneration, and more and more doctors are rallying to the cause. Because research is advancing so rapidly, this book can only be as up to date as our publication timeline allows. This chapter was last revised in August 1998. For research updates, please talk to your doctor, join the Association for Macular Diseases, or contact the Foundation Fighting Blindness or the Macular Degeneration Foundation. Their addresses and phone numbers are listed in the Appendices. You can also check our Web site at www.macularguide.com.

LASER

Laser is actually an acronym. It stands for **L**ight **A**mplification by **S**timulated **E**mission of **R**adiation. The name is confusing because it sounds like laser is an X ray, but as we know from movies, laser is an extremely fine beam of radiated light. Many patient brochures refer to "laser surgery," while others call it "laser treatment," but it's the same procedure either way. Laser for macular degeneration works on the abnormal blood vessels that develop with wet macular degeneration. Your ophthalmologist cauterizes each leaky blood vessel underneath the macula with laser, hopefully preventing the vessel from leaking any further. The procedure affects only the macula and the tissue underneath, leaving other areas of your eye untouched.

As a treatment option, laser has several big advantages. First, it is quick because the radiation beam takes only a fraction of a second to do its job. Also, laser is usually painless because your retina has no pain nerve endings, only visual nerve endings. And since the area of the macula that is treated has lost some of its ability to see, the laser's bright light is not usually irritating. Extensive laser treatment in a short period of time may cause discomfort and local anesthesia may be given, but most people with macular degeneration tolerate laser quite easily. Finally, laser is not incapacitating. The procedure is done in your ophthalmologist's office and requires no eye patches or special medicine regimen. You should be able to walk out minutes later and continue your daily routine.

Why Early Detection Is Important

Early detection of wet macular degeneration is necessary for laser to be effective. First of all, small problems are always easier to handle than large ones. So the fewer leaky blood vessels there are, the easier it is for the ophthalmologist to see them, and the better laser is able to seal them. More importantly, one of the great drawbacks of laser is that it usually cannot restore lost vision. When abnormal blood vessels grow and leak, they swamp patches of cone cells in the macula with blood, blocking the vision and usually causing these cells to die. Laser can stop the culprit blood vessel from leaking further, but it cannot revive dead cones. In some cases, though, people do experience slightly improved vision from laser when the blood pooling in their maculas drains away. It is important, therefore, to seal abnormal blood vessels when they threaten trouble, not after they have had plenty of time to bleed. Finally, laser can only be used on abnormal blood vessels that appear in the outer sections of the macula. If abnormal blood vessels are allowed to grow uncontrollably, they will eventually grow underneath the center of the macula, called the fovea. Your ophthalmologist cannot use laser on abnormal blood vessels underneath the fovea without risk of damage to the fovea itself, a problem explained in "The Laser Trade-Off" section below.

Early Detection: Using the Amsler Grid

Most patient brochures about ARMD reprint the Amsler Grid, so you may have seen it before. The Amsler Grid is designed to help you detect leaky, abnormal blood vessels caused by wet macular degeneration. By looking at the Amsler Grid with each eye separately, and noticing whether the appearance of the grid lines has changed, you may be able to tell whether or not new blood vessels are developing in your macula. Waviness in the lines, dark spots on the grid, or choppiness

HOW TO USE THE
AMSLER GRID

1. Put on your regular reading glasses. Cover your right eye. Use the same lighting each time.

2. Look only at the dot in the center of the grid.

3. If any lines around the dot are wavy, choppy, or distorted, or if a dark spot appears on the grid, tell your ophthalmologist immediately.

4. Cover your left eye and repeat the same steps.

are all typical distortions caused by a network of blood vessels under the retina. If they are detected early enough, your doctor may be able to treat these blood vessels with laser.

Because wet macular degeneration may develop from the dry form, many ophthalmologists give the Amsler Grid to all of their ARMD patients, even though laser is only useful for wet macular degeneration. Many brochures also suggest checking your vision daily. If you are experiencing early onset wet macular degeneration, this is sound

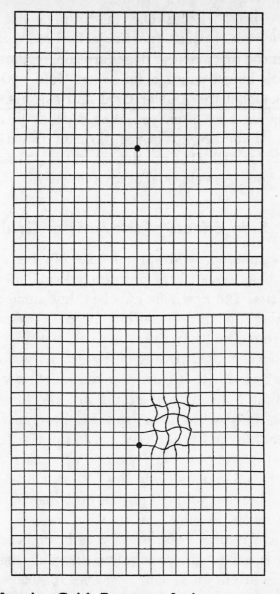

Top: Amsler Grid. Bottom: As it may appear to someone with early ARMD.

advice. But checking your vision daily is not necessary for many people, particularly those with very advanced dry macular degeneration, or those who are no longer eligible for laser. Talk with your doctor about the Amsler Grid and ask his or her advice on how often you should check your eyesight. If you are not in regular contact with your doctor for ARMD or another condition, you should have your eyes checked every two years.

Side Effects of the Amsler Grid

Unfortunately, widespread use of the Amsler Grid has caused three unintended side effects for patients. The first side effect is that some people feel terribly guilty once they discover their vision loss and find that there is such a thing as an Amsler Grid. "Why didn't I detect my vision loss right away?" Rosa Garcia asked me. "Now I find out that thousands of people are checking their vision daily, while I was running around without a clue! Maybe I could have saved my vision, but I wasn't paying careful enough attention." I am here to tell you, as I told Rosa, that it's really not fair to beat on yourself for not noticing changes in your vision.

As Chapter 1 discusses, your brain is actually hard-wired to ignore changes in your vision by paying attention to your best eye. If blood vessels develop slowly enough in one eye, you are unlikely to notice anything until they leak, causing the distortion or decrease in vision to become very pronounced. Until this happens, your brain will simply decide to see whatever it wants to see out of your other eye. In fact, you may not immediately notice changes in your vision even if you cover each eye and check with an Amsler Grid. That's because our visual system is also designed to fill in whatever information seems missing when we look at something. Sometimes your brain will tell you that you see a complete Amsler Grid, even when your eyes are actually perceiving wavy lines. This is a wonderful evolutionary adaptation for an era before laser, although it isn't a great advantage in this one situation. But that is not your fault.

The second unintended side effect is that some people find checking the Amsler Grid daily very stressful. You are very unlikely to get out of bed, sit with one hand over your right eye, peer at the Amsler Grid, and discover that your vision has improved. So checking the Amsler Grid is like asking whether today is the same as yesterday or worse. It's an exercise in looking for the negative. That's one reason why it's worth asking your doctor whether or not checking the Amsler Grid daily is necessary.

Finally, the third side effect of the Amsler Grid is that it is often the only thing patients receive from their doctors or from brochures. This gives many people the impression that the Amsler Grid is the only tool available. You stick it on your refrigerator, and then what? While a wonderful test, the Amsler Grid has very limited application. It is useful for facilitating early laser treatments that are effective in a small percentage of patients. That's it. It can't provide visual rehabilitation, emotional coping strategies, marital counseling for vision loss, or information on nutrition or research. It's just a little grid. And people with macular degeneration need a whole lot more than a little grid.

The Laser Trade-Off

"We had an informational open house for people with macular degeneration," a prominent physician recently admitted to me, "and it was crazy. There were one hundred seniors in the audience. Half of them were waving their hands and shouting 'I had doctor so-and-so who did four lasers on my eye and now I'm blind! No one explained to me what would happen! I signed a consent form but no one told me it would get worse! They did this laser surgery and I was better off before!' The other half were holding onto their chairs and shouting 'Sit down and let the doctor finish!' I could hardly get a word in edgewise. One of the retinal specialists on our panel went to get a glass of water. He was mobbed. He came running back up to the podium and asked, 'Is there a back door in this building?'"

Clearly, laser doesn't leave a lot of people

happy, even those who detected their wet macular degeneration early. Why not? As I mentioned, the first limitation of laser is that it usually doesn't restore vision. Many people hear this from their doctors before their laser, but it is impossible not to hope for better vision afterward, so many people do, and they are disappointed. What laser does best is prevent *additional* vision loss caused by existing abnormal blood vessels. Secondly, laser is helpful in only 7 percent of macular degeneration cases. About 10 percent to 15 percent of the people who have macular degeneration have the type of wet macular degeneration that is eligible for laser. Laser delays vision loss in 70 percent of the people who receive it. However, 50 percent of this group have recurrent bleeding later on, because new abnormal blood vessels grow or old ones reopen.

But the biggest drawback of laser, which many people do not fully understand before they undergo treatment, is what I call the "blind spot for better vision trade-off." When a laser beam hits an abnormal blood vessel underneath the macula, the heat of the beam burns a tiny scar in the macula itself, causing a small blind spot, which is noticeable to many patients. This is why abnormal blood vessels right underneath the fovea, the center of the macula, are not as amenable to laser. It's arguably a sensible trade-off to get a small blind spot to the side of your central vision in order to preserve the rest of your central vision, but lasering a vessel underneath the fovea can put a blind spot right in the center of your vision. In spite of this, however, laser has been proven to reduce the severity of vision loss in some people when applied to the fovea.

So what does this blind spot look like? Before laser, you may see blurry images or gray in the area affected by an abnormal blood vessel. After laser you may see a darker spot in that same area. This dark spot may seem more pronounced than blurry images or gray, so it really bothers some people. Certainly, it's a shock if it's not expected. Some people, however, do not notice a particular dark spot, although they may notice that their vision is not quite as good as it was before. If you don't receive laser, however, the abnormal blood vessels causing your vision loss may extend all the way underneath the macula and continue bleeding. Once they do, they will cause dark or gray areas in the center of your vision all by themselves. By that time, they cannot be lasered without damaging your macula further. So both patient and ophthalmologist are in a dilemma: if no treatment is offered, the patient's vision is likely to deteriorate rapidly. If laser is applied, the patient's vision will deteriorate more slowly, but the patient may immediately experience a dark spot. As Neil Bressler, M.D., of Johns Hopkins University puts it, with laser "you are giving someone poor vision to prevent terrible vision."

Is Laser Right for You?

Now that you know about the "blind spot for better vision trade-off," you can make a more informed choice with your doctor about laser. Many people, however, are not eligible for this approach. Lasers can treat only wet macular degeneration, not dry. If you have the wet type, you have either "classic" or "occult" subretinal neovascular membranes (SRNV), also called choroidal neovascularization (CNV), or a combination of both types. Classic wet ARMD is called "classic" because it was discovered first, is easier to detect, and is more familiar to doctors. Laser was developed to treat classic CNV, and all research on laser is based on classic CNV. Occult CNV is a different bird. It has subtler blood vessel patterns, is much harder to identify, and was discovered very recently. We don't yet know very much about it, including whether or not laser would be effective in treating it. Therefore, as of now, you are eligible for laser only if you have classic wet macular degeneration. It is possible, however, to have both classic and occult CNV. Some researchers believe that undetected occult CNV may be responsible for the high rate of recurrent bleeding that many people experience after their laser for classic CNV.

Experiencing Angiograms and Laser

Once you have detected changes in your vision, and your doctor believes that you may have classic pattern wet ARMD, what happens next? Generally, you will have a fluorescein angiogram anywhere from a few minutes to a few days before your laser. Fluorescein is a type of dye, and an angiogram is a type of photograph that shows dye in blood vessels. Fluorescein angiograms allow your doctor to see the blood vessels in your eye much more clearly and to determine the risk of damage to your macula and the feasibility of laser. Fluorescein angiograms are common and painless (except for one quick needle prick in your arm). The vast majority of people experience no side effects; occasionally someone may become nauseated or develop hives, and rarely a serious allergic reaction occurs. Your doctor can do one in the office. When you have a fluorescein angiogram, your doctor or technician will inject dye into your arm. The dye travels very quickly throughout your blood vessels, including the abnormal ones in your eye, making them much more visible. Then the technician will take flash photographs of your eye. It's very simple.

Fluorescein angiograms reveal classic pattern wet macular degeneration. Your doctor may recommend an indocyanine green angiogram, also called an ICG, if it is suspected that an occult vessel pattern is present. An ICG is just like a fluorescein angiogram, except it uses a different type of dye that allows your doctor to see more complex, subtle blood vessels more easily. Sometimes both dyes may be injected at the same time, enabling your doctor to do both types of angiograms in a single appointment.

Like angiograms, laser can be done in just a few minutes in your ophthalmologist's office. To prepare for laser, your doctor will dilate your pupils with drops, just as if you were having a regular checkup, and may inject numbing medication near the eye to prevent eye movement during the treatment. Then you simply rest your chin and forehead against supports, and look straight ahead. Your doctor uses a tiny red aiming beam to guide the laser. A laser beam takes only a fraction of a second to cauterize a blood vessel in your eye, although if there are a lot of vessels to cauterize, a treatment may take fifteen to twenty minutes. That's it. Aside from having dilated pupils and being a little more sensitive to light for a while, you will be able to walk out minutes later with no difficulty. You may immediately notice the small blind spot from the laser described above, or your vision may clear somewhat if the blood pooling in your macula drains after the blood vessels are cauterized. Many people, however, do not notice much of a difference. Remember, if you have glaucoma or cataracts, the laser will not affect either condition, so vision loss from these two conditions will not be restored.

CATARACT SURGERY AND MACULAR DEGENERATION

Just as many people are less than pleased with laser, many of my ARMD patients have been less than pleased with their cataract surgery. Why? The first reason is that many people logically expect to see much more clearly after cataract surgery than they did before. If you have advancing macular degeneration, however, your cataract surgery will probably give you more overall light perception and make things brighter by removing your old cloudy lenses, but it may not give you clearer vision. Macular degeneration may be blurring your central vision regardless of your cataracts, and cataract surgery cannot solve that problem. Be hopeful, but also be realistic about what cataract surgery can and can't do.

Secondly, many patients have remarked that they do not see as well after their cataract surgery as they did before. Why? It may be possible that cataract surgery aggravates macular degeneration. If this turns out to be true, it's an entirely new finding that is not now commonly accepted. But there are two studies that seem to suggest exactly this. The Beaver Dam Eye Study observed that people who have had cataract surgery are more likely to have early macular degeneration than people who haven't, but it did not find a correlation between cataract surgery and advanced macular degeneration. One possible explanation is that early ARMD is easier to detect after dense cataracts are removed, meaning that cataract surgery doesn't cause but simply allows us to detect macular degeneration more easily.

On the other hand, a 1996 Israeli study does show an increased rate of wet macular degeneration after cataract surgery, particularly in men. If this is true, there are several reasons why this might occur. The most persuasive may be that the loss of pressure in the eye during cataract surgery when the lens is removed and replaced may aggravate the abnormal blood vessels in your macula. All researchers have called for additional studies, which we will need before we have a firm understanding of the relationship between cataract surgery and ARMD. In the meantime, if you have concerns, discuss them with your doctor.

WHY MEDICAL PROGRESS SEEMS SO SLOW

Why does progress in this area seem so slow? The first reason may lie in the condition itself. Because ARMD affects seniors instead of children or midlife adults, it's very difficult to collect data on inheritance patterns. The parents of most seniors with macular degeneration today have already passed away, so we cannot know for sure whether they had it, too. The children of most seniors with ARMD will not develop the condition for another ten to thirty years. And there is no way to predict which of these adult children may develop the condition and which will not. By comparison, heart attacks and cancer affect people in much wider age ranges, so it's easier to gather more information about the trends of these conditions.

Secondly, degenerative conditions are notoriously more difficult to treat than acute conditions, no matter where they occur in the body. Degenerative conditions tend to be harder to fix through surgery or drugs, and Western medicine is very surgery and drug focused. It's a whole lot easier to deal with a cataract, for example, than to know what to do with macular degeneration because cataracts are opacities of the lens sitting on the front of your eye. They can easily be surgically removed and replaced with artificial lens implants. Macular degeneration, on the other hand, affects several different layers of irreplaceable tissue underneath your retina, way in the back of your eye. Just getting to the area can be a challenge. Unlike replacing a hip or fixing a broken bone, degenerative conditions are often chronic, and it's very difficult to get to the root of chronic conditions, at least with modern medicine. We never quite fix the problem; we simply wind up treating symptoms. In this case, cauterizing an abnormal blood vessel with laser stops that particular vessel, but that vessel is really a symptom of the larger condition. Laser doesn't treat the possible causes or prevent new blood vessels from growing.

Thirdly, any new treatment for macular degeneration needs to be thoroughly studied before it is approved. This is not just a matter of avoiding law suits or jumping through hoops for the federal government. Federal standards regulating the use of new treatments are designed to protect your overall health as well as your pocketbook. Some doctors and many patients find it tempting to use an experimental treatment "just in case it works" or because "there's nothing to lose." But there is a possibility that unproven treatments may cause more harm than good. Even if experimental therapies cause no harm, they may be ineffective and leave you with large medical bills. So new treatments, especially those that may be dangerous, need to be tested through large, long-term, controlled, randomized, and double-masked studies before they are made available to patients.

Whoa! What does all that mean? "Controlled studies" are those that compare people who receive an experimental treatment with people who receive no treatment to insure that the treatment is actually making a positive difference. "Randomized" means that participants are assigned randomly to either the treated or the nontreated group. If you don't randomize a study, you are likely to get skewed results because you may wind up putting all the participants with better or worse vision in a particular group. Finally, "double-masked studies" are those in which neither the participants nor the experimenters know who is in the treated group and who is in the untreated group. This strategy is necessary to avoid bias on the part of the researchers and a false sense of improvement or failure on the part of the participants. As you can guess, these studies are expensive and take a lot of time to design and complete. Additionally, studies that are large enough to produce conclusive results require the participation and cooperation of many research centers.

As of today, the only treatment for macular degeneration that has been proven effective and safe in a controlled, randomized study is laser for classic wet macular degeneration. But we eagerly await the results of studies in progress worldwide.

ONGOING RESEARCH AND RESULTS

Macular degeneration is an international problem. The lack of effective medical options has spurred research for new treatments in many countries. Doctors and scientists are working on a wide range of options, including new forms of laser, radiation treatments, surgery, and drugs. Patients are beginning to track research results as they eagerly await a breakthrough, especially in Scandinavia, where macular degeneration is very common. "Patients now come to my office with fifty printed papers in hand," Finnish low-vision specialist Dr. Lea Hyvärinen told me recently. "They've already investigated what's happening in America and in other countries. They say, 'I got on the Internet and this is what I found. Now I would like you to go home and think about it.'" The media have begun to pay more attention to macular degeneration studies, too. Unfortunately, the media sometimes report research results prematurely or incompletely, causing public confusion. In order to clarify the status of recent research up to August 1998, I have summarized all of the major medical treatment studies below, except for nutrition studies, which are discussed in the next chapter. Updates will be posted on our Web site: www.macularguide.com.

EXPERIMENTAL FORMS OF LASER

One of the biggest problems with laser is the damage it may do to the macula as a result of the heat of the laser beam. To solve this problem, researchers are experimenting with Photodynamic Therapy (PDT), an attempt to use a low-intensity nonthermal (non–heat producing) laser. Julia Levy, Ph.D., of the University of British Columbia, whose mother has macular degeneration, came up with the idea. It's really rather ingenious. The procedure relies on taking free radicals, which we normally think of as bad, and using them to our advantage. (See Chapter 3 for a discussion of free radicals and ARMD.) It begins by injecting a photosensitizing dye into the patient's arm, just as if he or she were having an angiogram. When the dye collects in the abnormal blood vessels of the macula, the vessels are lasered, causing the dye to react with the vessel tissue. This reaction produces free radicals. The free radicals, in turn, act to close off the unwanted vessels and prevent further leaking.

EXPERIMENTAL RADIATION TREATMENT

Researchers in Europe and the United States are now testing whether or not general radiation exposure, rather than focused laser beams, will inhibit the growth of abnormal blood vessels in the eye without damaging it. The results so far are encouraging but inconclusive. The published studies have been preliminary in nature, and none of them have used reliable enough research procedures to draw firm conclusions. Some researchers have found that their patients' vision improved, others found no effect, and still others have found that their patients' vision improved briefly and then declined again. There are now three major studies underway in the U.S., the Netherlands, and the U.K. on large numbers of patients with standardized doses of radiation, randomized control groups, and double-blind evaluation of effects, so solid knowledge will be forthcoming.

Unfortunately, some radiologists are treating desperate macular degeneration patients, sometimes without even checking their vision before and after the radiation treatment. Since patients do not see a new blind spot immediately after radiation therapy, as they often do after laser treatment, and since results are not expected for up to a year, patients tend to be satisfied with radiation therapy. But their vision may in fact be no different several months after radiation treatment than it was before; it may in fact be deteriorating more rapidly after radiation than if they had not been treated. This is one risk of accepting an experimental treatment that has not been adequately studied. As a result, ophthalmologists at the 1997 International Symposium on Radiation Therapy for Macular Degeneration called for a moratorium on radiation treatments except within the context of approved, controlled clinical studies with sufficient follow-up time. This declaration was reemphasized at the 1998 Johns Hopkins University/Foundation Fighting Blindness Symposium on Macular Degeneration.

EXPERIMENTAL SURGERIES

Retinal Rotation, Retinal Shift, or Macular Translocation

As we know, when the abnormal blood vessels of wet macular degeneration grow directly under the fovea, which is the center of the macula, laser treatments are not possible without damaging the fovea itself. To get around this problem, Robert Machemer, M.D., of Duke University, began experimenting with moving the fovea a few millimeters by cutting a big circle in the retina, loosening it from the tissue below, and rotating it so the fovea sits atop an area without abnormal blood vessels. This procedure is called retinal rotation, retinal shift, or macular translocation. Once the fovea has been rotated, Dr. Machemer applies laser treatments to cauterize the abnormal vessels where the fovea was originally. At Johns Hopkins University, Eugene DeJuan, Jr., M.D., revised this technique to allow for smaller, safer incisions. In Japan, Yasuo Tano, M.D., has done experimental surgeries based on Dr. Machemer and Dr. DeJuan's work, and in Germany

Claus Eckart, M.D., has also developed an original technique for the same surgery.

Macular translocation surgery is feasible for only a limited number of people and there are still real risks of retinal detachment, which causes severe vision loss, and of underrotating the fovea, which eliminates the benefit of the surgery altogether. In addition, if the fovea is moved and any vision is in fact restored, the world will appear titled at an unnatural angle. To overcome this, Dr. Eckart performs eye muscle surgery along with the retinal surgery. Time and much more research will tell whether these surgeries will prove to be sight-saving, but both Dr. Eckart and Dr. DeJuan are sufficiently encouraged by their results to continue testing and refining their procedures.

Submacular Surgery

Submacular surgery is an alternative to macular translocation. Instead of moving the fovea to someplace that doesn't have abnormal blood vessels underneath, the goal is to remove the abnormal blood vessels themselves, a technique first described by Matthew Thomas, M.D., of St. Louis. Michael Lambert, M.D., at Baylor College of Medicine in Texas operated on forty-nine patients with wet macular degeneration and reported that 50 percent experienced somewhat improved vision. He also found that only 12 percent experienced new abnormal blood vessel growth in the areas in which he had operated. Dr. Thomas subsequently reported limited, if any, improvements in a large group of patients with ARMD, and physicians at the Kresge Eye Institute in Detroit noted that 40 percent of their patients experienced new abnormal blood vessel growth within two years after this surgery. In the least encouraging study, twenty patients underwent the same surgery at the University of Toronto, Canada, with very little improvement in vision. Nearly 50 percent of these patients had new abnormal blood vessels in the same area within twelve months after surgery.

We are currently awaiting the results of the Subfoveal Surgery Trial sponsored by the National Eye Institute that should determine the effectiveness of this surgery. In the meantime, researchers continue to refine submacular surgery techniques. They are also looking into the possibility of combining it with cell transplants to restore vision.

Submacular Surgery with t-PA

Chapter 1 explains how bleeding from abnormal blood vessels in wet macular degeneration floods the cones of the macula, depriving them of oxygen. There is another problem with uncontrolled bleeding in the macula. Fibrin, which causes our blood to clot when we start bleeding, gets stuck between cone cells like globs of superglue, squishing the cone cells together and distorting their shape. These superglue clots of fibrin are nearly impossible to remove surgically without damaging the cones themselves. Fibrin clots also make submacular surgery much harder and less successful. To solve this problem, Hilel Lewis, M.D., of the Cleveland Clinic, and other researchers are studying the effectiveness of injecting the fibrin-dissolving drug tissue plasminogen activator (t-PA) into clotted areas during submacular surgery. Initial results from clinical studies show that t-PA may be very helpful for those people with early stage wet macular degeneration and only very recent bleeding, but more studies are needed to assess t-PA's effectiveness.

Transplants

"What I need is a whole new eye," Buddy Burmester once joked, half seriously. We don't have the technology right now to transplant eyes, but some researchers believe we will in the next century. We can, however, transplant parts of eyes, like corneas. Researchers at many hospitals and universities are now trying to figure out how to transplant cells in the tissue underneath the macula in order to rejuvenate the macula's support system. The idea is to introduce new cells that will grow healthy replacement parts, just like bone marrow transplants encourage new marrow growth. Two types of cells are used in these experiments:

retinal pigment epithelium (RPE) cells, and cone and rod cells from the macula itself.

We know that these cells can be transplanted and grow, but we don't yet know if they will then actually improve vision. In addition, the likelihood that our own eyes would reject transplant cells is still an unsolved problem. Clearly, transplant surgery is still at a very early stage of research and will not be available even for voluntary clinical trials for some time. Finally, the best source of RPE cells is fetal eyes, because cells from fetal eyes are likely to have a higher potential to proliferate and grow than cells from any other source, including our own eyes. Fetal cells are also less likely to be rejected by the recipient's immune system. Using eyes from human fetuses for research is controversial, however, and some people may not want to accept fetal transplants.

EXPERIMENTAL DRUG TREATMENTS

Interferon

Interferon is a substance made in laboratories and by the body to interfere with viruses. For a while, interferon injections seemed to prevent the growth of unwanted blood vessels in wet macular degeneration. Excited by these reports, researchers at forty-five eye centers worldwide conducted a randomized, controlled, double-masked study on interferon, providing the highest level of research accuracy possible. By 1997, though, they concluded that interferon is not effective. Their results showed no significant difference between study participants who took interferon and those who did not. In fact, the study participants who took the highest doses of interferon wound up with worse vision than those who took no interferon. The bad news is that interferon is not helpful. The good news is that now these researchers are pursuing other leads, and a great deal of information was yielded through this study about the natural course of macular degeneration. The interferon study also illustrates the value of a large, controlled study for determining the effectiveness of treatments.

Thalidomide

The name thalidomide brings chills to most of us who remember the disfiguring birth defects it caused in the 1950s when it was prescribed to treat morning sickness. Hundreds of babies affected by thalidomide failed to grow normal arms or legs. The thalidomide tragedy now stands in medical history as a classic example of the folly of prescribing drugs before they have been thoroughly tested. Since the 1950s, however, we've discovered that thalidomide also inhibits the growth of blood vessels in animal eyes. Perhaps this drug, which has caused so much pain to so many people, may provide relief, too. It may also inhibit the growth of unwanted blood vessels in wet macular degeneration.

To test this hypothesis, Allen C. Ho, M.D., of the Scheie Institute of the University of Pennsylvania, is coordinating a pilot study called **A**ge-related **M**acular **D**egeneration **A**nd **T**halidomide **S**tudy (AMDATS). He hopes to determine the value of thalidomide treatment itself, and to see if taking thalidomide after laser treatments would increase the effectiveness of the laser. Two groups of patients are currently participating in his study. If the results are positive, a larger study conducted at several sites around the country will follow. Thalidomide is a very powerful drug that may have as yet unknown side effects. Experience warns us that careful and complete trials are necessary before distributing the drug for widespread use.

VEGF

In the 1940s, scientists suggested that retinal cells that do not receive enough oxygen may produce a chemical substance to stimulate the development of blood vessels in the retina. We now believe that **V**ascular **E**ndothelial **G**rowth **F**actor (VEGF) may be that chemical substance. This means that all those unwanted blood vessels that grow because of wet macular degeneration may be triggered by the retina itself or the RPE. If this is true, then antibodies to VEGF may stop VEGF from being produced, and thereby stop new blood vessel growth.

Joan Miller, M.D., of the Massachusetts Eye and Ear Infirmary and Harvard Medical School, and her colleagues have shown in their laboratory that VEGF is present during the development of new vessels, that it is produced by both retinal and RPE cells when these cells lack oxygen, and that it is undetectable in animal eyes that have not experienced a lack of oxygen. They have also shown that VEGF injections into normal animal eyes can produce new vessel growth, which can be prevented by injections of antibodies to VEGF.

Dr. Miller's findings are exciting. They also raise several important questions. For example, is there a certain amount of VEGF that we need in our eyes to maintain our normal blood vessels or other retinal functions? How can we make sure that if we inject antibodies they will affect only abnormal new blood vessels and not the ones we need? Would injections of antibodies to VEGF be toxic to people in some way? Dr. Miller and others are now trying to answer these questions. A clinical trial of VEGF is also under way in Sweden.

Integrin Antagonists

Integrin are little molecules that act as taxi drivers for other cells in our bodies. They help other molecules, including VEGF, navigate and do their jobs. Martin Friedlander, M.D., of Scripps Research Institute has already shown that new blood vessel growth can be inhibited in animal eyes by using drugs, commonly called integrin antagonists, that neutralize integrin. Once these drugs neutralize integrin, integrin can't help VEGF move around to different cells, and VEGF can't stimulate abnormal blood vessel growth. The next step is to determine whether we can get the same results in human eyes.

THE FUTURE

Some prominent physicians, like David Guyer, M.D., of Manhattan Eye and Ear Hospital, believe that improvements in laser technology and drug research for macular degeneration provide the most promising leads. In the not-so-distant future, we may be able to offer cool low-power laser treatments to cauterize wet macular degeneration blood vessels without damaging the macula, along with prescription medications to prevent recurring blood vessel growth.

In addition to these advancements in surgery and drug treatments for ARMD, researchers are exploring new methods of prevention, which is certainly the best long term solution. For example, Wyeth-Ayerst Pharmaceuticals is currently investigating the effects of estrogen, a powerful antioxidant, on macular degeneration. They expect to show by 2005 that estrogen replacement therapy may help reduce ARMD. In the meantime, though, there are things we can reasonably do today to minimize our risk of macular degeneration.

CHAPTER 3

Genes and Greens:
The Causes and Prevention
of ARMD

It sounds funny to recommend
spinach, given the sophistication of
modern medicine, but there's ample,
basic scientific evidence that shows it
is important to the eyes.
Physicians might do patients a
service by prescribing cookbooks.
—Stuart Richter, O.D., Ph.D.

Mother Nature is no less difficult or
more complicated than any other
mother.
—John Breitner, M.D., M.P.H.
Johns Hopkins School
of Hygiene and Public Health

No one yet understands exactly what causes
macular degeneration. There probably isn't one
single big cause but rather a combination of

smaller causes that accumulate to trigger the condition. What we do understand from demographic studies is who is more likely to get ARMD and what characteristics they share. These two sets of information allow us to make reasonable judgments about what may cause macular degeneration. And it allows us to report risk factors and recommend things you can do to minimize your risk of advanced macular degeneration.

Rod and Cone Cell Damage: Two Possible Sources

As you may recall from Chapter 1, macular degeneration is basically a breakdown of the support tissue conveyor-belt system maintaining the rod and cone cells of the macula. In dry macular degeneration, the support tissues find themselves unable to flush away damaged metabolic waste products from the rods and cones. As a result, deposits of waste and lipids accumulate, clogging the system and preventing proper oxygen flow to the cells. Eventually, the rods and cones asphyxiate. In wet macular degeneration, weak abnormal blood vessels grow through the support tissues. These vessels leak, flooding the cones and asphyxiating them. To put it in greater detail, there seem to be two possible scenarios that explain how macular degeneration occurs:

1. Damaged metabolic waste build-up

In this scenario the culprit is damaged or abnormal waste. Rod and cone cells have disposable lipid (fatty) tips. When they process light and metabolize oxygen, the tips fall off as waste and new tips grow. Normally these tips are collected by the RPE and transported down a few layers on the conveyor belt to waiting blood vessels, which flush the tips into the bloodstream. But damaged waste tips lack the handles the RPE uses to identify them and drag them away, so they sit around accumulating like little chunks of cement, making it difficult for the RPE to clear away additional waste or deliver more oxygen. The lack of oxygen first kills the RPE, then the rods and cones, and may trigger the growth of abnormal, leaky blood vessels that characterize wet macular degeneration.

2. Poor blood vessel health and performance

In this scenario, the blood vessels supporting the macula's maintenance system do not deliver oxygen quickly enough or pick up waste efficiently enough. As a result, the rods and cones and the underlying tissue lack adequate oxygen and become clogged with waste. The lack of oxygen kills the RPE, and then the rod and cone cells, and may trigger the growth of the abnormal, leaky blood vessels that characterize wet macular degeneration.

The question now becomes: What is causing the rod and cone cells to produce abnormal waste tips? And what is causing poor blood vessel performance and health? For answers, we need to turn to the characteristics that many people with macular degeneration have in common.

LEADING RISK FACTORS

The biggest characteristic that people with ARMD share is age. You are more likely to develop macular degeneration at seventy-five than at sixty, probably because the support system for your macula has had fifteen more years to become overwhelmed, and your blood vessels may be less healthy and vigorous. As a result, more women have macular degeneration than men, because more women live longer. Besides age, there are four more characteristics that many people with macular degeneration have in common: smoking,

---

THE LEADING RISK FACTORS FOR ARMD

1. Smoking
2. Family history
3. Diet low in dark green leafy vegetables
4. Blue or light-colored eyes
5. Sun exposure or low sun tolerance

---

a family history of macular degeneration, a diet low in dark green leafy vegetables, and blue or light-colored eyes. These four characteristics are the first four risk factors for ARMD. In other words, if you have any of these factors, your risk of developing macular degeneration is greater than if you don't. How much greater? We aren't sure, but greater nonetheless. However, these risk factors are not a guarantee. You can find people with blue eyes who have avoided dark green leafy vegetables all their lives and don't have macular degeneration. You can find people with dark brown eyes who have never smoked and do have macular degeneration. But these are exceptions and thus harder to find than those who fit the risk profile.

There is one last leading risk factor: sun exposure without blue light protection, especially in people with fair skin or light eyes. Since very few people in the United States have ever consistently worn sunglasses with blue blockers, which provide blue light protection, we assume that everyone has this risk factor. Why is it on the list? Because there is increasing evidence that blue light damages the macula, and may increase the volume of waste that accumulates in your eye with dry macular degeneration. To understand how this could happen, and why the first four risk factors may also contribute to waste accumulation in the macula and poor blood vessel health and performance, you need to understand a little bit about free radicals and antioxidants.

FREE RADICALS AND ANTIOXIDANTS

Free radicals are oxygen molecules with an electron missing, which makes them unstable. Left to their own devices, free radicals cause trouble by reacting with other molecules in our bodies, preventing them from doing their jobs or actually destabilizing their structures. You may have heard of free radicals lately, since they are now believed to play an important role in the development of certain cancers. Free radicals are a normal part of our system. We produce them as byproducts of oxygen metabolism. We metabolize a lot of oxygen in our maculas, so we produce a lot of free radicals there. Mother Nature has provided our bodies with a natural mechanism for handling free radicals. They are usually picked up and carried off by antioxidants, molecules we get from our food that are designed to pair up electrically with free radicals and neutralize them. So we are actually designed to handle a certain amount of naturally occurring free radicals. If this is true, though, why are free radicals a problem?

The problem is that pesticides, pollution, car exhaust, cigarette smoke, and excessive unprotected sun exposure, which we wind up eating, breathing, and soaking up in record amounts, also produce free radicals. These free radicals are toxic to our eyes and bodies. They overwhelm our limited supply of antioxidants, especially if we aren't replenishing our antioxidants by eating foods that contain them. When this happens, free radicals are literally free to react with the lipids in the cones of our macula, producing abnormal waste tips. It is thought that these waste tips don't have normal waste labels or handles, or even normal waste consistency, so they can't be grabbed and processed by the RPE. Instead, they accumulate in permanent deposits, backing up the conveyor belt until it can't process any more waste or deliver any more oxygen for that particular area. It's essentially the equivalent of putting cement blocks in a garbage disposal. Nothing happens to the blocks, but the disposal breaks.

The Environment Is a Major Source of Free Radicals

We are just beginning to understand how what we produce in our environment, and what we eat and breathe affect our health. Cancer, some birth defects, asthma, allergies, and other autoimmune conditions have been linked to industrial pollution of one kind or another. There is still much research to do on the many unanswered questions, but it looks more and more as if macular degeneration may join this list, making environmental regulations and adequate diets critically important. For our overall health we should demand that legislators protect our air and water, and we should protect our bodies by eating well. Macular degeneration is appearing in other industrialized areas of the world, which suggests that environmental factors may be even more important than a family history of the condition. Japan has reported increasing numbers of cases, and ARMD is becoming common in South America. Conversely, there is some evidence that people who live in nonpolluted, rural areas with fresh food may have less risk of macular degeneration. One 1997 study conducted in the isolated, nonindustrial mountain village of Salandra, Italy, where residents grew their own food, found that even though 30 percent of the population had blue eyes, their rate of macular degeneration was less than half the American rate reported by the Beaver Dam Eye Study.

What About Genetics?

If our environment is so important, why does it increase your risk to have a family history of macular degeneration? In the United States, ARMD appears to cluster in families, although there is no clear inheritance pattern—from father to son, for example, or mother to daughter. We do not yet understand the interplay of environmental influences and genetics with this condition. Some people may be genetically more susceptible to free radicals, or genes may sometimes play a larger role in the development of ARMD than we now understand. In fact, some researchers, like Edwin M. Stone, M.D., of the University of Iowa, are working to prove that ARMD is one of a group of inherited disorders. He is also supported by fellow researchers, Paulus deJon, M.D., Ph.D., of the Netherlands, who calculates that 23 percent of ARMD may be attributed to a genetic component, and Johanna Seddon, M.D., of Harvard University, who has found that people who have relatives with macular degeneration are three times more likely to develop the condition than those who do not. However, we have yet to fully understand the genetics of ARMD.

In 1997, a team of researchers reported that 16 percent of people with macular degeneration, particularly dry macular degeneration, share a mutation in their ABCR gene. ABCR stands for **A**TP **B**inding **C**assette **R**etina transporter gene. This same mutation was found to cause Stargardt's disease, the juvenile form of macular degeneration, by researchers supported by the Foundation Fighting Blindness (FFB). Researchers are now asking whether ABCR plays a role in our retina's waste management system by enabling the transportation of various molecules. If it does, and if the ABCR gene is defective, then waste material would build up in the retina and the

RPE, eventually damaging the conveyor belt system that supports the macula. Researchers hoped this would turn out to be the case, because transporter genes like ABCR are very amenable to drug treatments, which compensate for the gene's poor performance, or gene therapy, which replaces the defective gene with a healthy one.

In 1998, however, Dr. Stone conducted a study of 182 people with ARMD, 206 with Stargardt's disease, and 96 controls (people who have neither condition). He screened every single ABCR gene of every single person. He found 1,100 ABCR gene variations, but not a single variant was more common in people with ARMD than in the others. There was no statistical evidence in his study that an ABCR gene defect causes macular degeneration. Dr. Stone concluded that great caution is required in assigning the cause of ARMD to any particular gene. We may eventually find a genetic cause, but it may be more complicated than finding a single gene.

WHAT YOU CAN DO TO REDUCE YOUR RISK

There are four things you can do to reduce your overload of free radicals and increase your chances of avoiding advanced macular degeneration. First, don't smoke and avoid second-hand smoke. Second, wear sunglasses with blue blockers, and finally, eat a balanced low-fat diet high in antioxidants for the macula, and take a balanced dose of vitamins and minerals. That's the whole ball game in a nutshell. Why shouldn't you smoke?

REDUCE YOUR RISK

1. Do not smoke. Avoid second-hand smoke.

2. Wear sunglasses with blue blockers.

3. Eat a *balanced*, natural, low-fat diet with five servings per week of dark green leafy vegetables. Eat organic produce whenever possible.

4. Take a *balanced*, reasonable dose of vitamins and minerals.

What are blue blockers? Which vegetables are high in antioxidants for the macula? Can eating right slow the development of macular degeneration once you already have it? What vitamins should you take? The rest of this chapter will answer these questions, explain the top four recommendations for reducing your risk of ARMD in greater detail, and outline the current research on its causes and prevention.

A word of caution before you continue reading: always check with your doctor before changing your diet or exercise habits. You may have health conditions or medications that will require modifying these recommendations, especially if you smoke, have high blood pressure, heart disease, diabetes, or are taking coumadin. Eating excessive amounts of spinach may affect your thyroid, so vary your vegetable intake and remember to eat a balanced low-fat diet.

1. Stop Smoking

No one should smoke. If you don't smoke, don't start. If you do smoke, stop now. I know that quitting is incredibly difficult, and smoking is a great pleasure. But smoking is terrible for your health, and for the health of anyone who breathes your smoke. Smoking contributes to cancer, heart disease, emphysema, asthma, and apparently macular degeneration. Smoking adversely affects blood circulation and blood vessel health, making wet macular degeneration more likely. And smoking overloads your eyes with free radicals, using up the lutein, zeaxanthin, and vitamins C and E your eyes need to take care of the naturally occurring free radicals produced by oxygen consumption in the macula. Smoking also inhibits vitamins from being processed. I can't say enough bad things about smoking, and I can't think of anything good about it, especially not for your eyes. If you must smoke, it is doubly important that you follow the remaining recommendations for reducing your risk of macular degeneration, especially the diet and vitamin recommendations.

2. Wear Sunglasses with Blue Blockers

You are probably already aware of the importance of wearing sunglasses with ultraviolet (UV) light protection. UV light waves are invisible to us, but they can contribute to cataracts. Opticians add UV protection to the prescription sunglasses they sell, and many over-the-counter brands have UV protection, too. You can request UV protection in your clear glasses since it will not add tint. It turns out, however, the UV light rays are not the only ones that may cause damage to our eyes. Extensive laboratory studies of primates provide persuasive evidence that blue light may be even more damaging to the macula than UV light.

Blue Light and Macular Degeneration

In many primate studies, blue light has been shown to cause a photochemical reaction that produces free radicals in the RPE and the rods and cones. Researchers believe that these free radicals interact with the high oxygen and lipid content in human rod and cone tips to produce abnormal chunks of metabolized waste that cannot be properly processed by the RPE, clogging up the macula's maintenance system and producing dry macular degeneration.

Melanin, the substance that gives eyes their color, protects the macula by trapping light rays so they don't reach the macula and cause damage. People with fair skin and blue or light-colored eyes may be particularly susceptible to macular damage by blue light because they have less melanin in their irises. Their blue eyes transmit up to one hundred times as much light to the back of the eye as dark colored eyes do. Additionally, when the light reaches the choroid and RPE of people with fair skin and blue eyes, there is less melanin there to absorb the radiant energy, leaving these tissues more vulnerable to light damage. Can blue light rays cause macular degeneration? Can you reduce your risk by protecting your eyes from blue light? The answer is maybe.

Although the laboratory studies on animals seem nearly unanimous, the real world studies on people have produced conflicting results. Some studies positively link macular degeneration with any kind of light exposure, other studies have found a weak correlation between macular degeneration and blue light exposure, and yet a third group of studies has found no correlation at all between macular degeneration and sunlight. One Australian study concluded that the problem is not total sun exposure, but exactly how sensitive you are to the sun. It hypothesized that people who have plenty of melanin and don't tend to burn easily are at less risk for macular degeneration than people who burn easily or are bothered by sun glare. This study also concluded that people with blue irises are at increased risk for ARMD. These results, which have not been replicated or confirmed, do not allow me to state absolutely that blue light contributes to the development of macular degeneration, but it is certainly plausible. Based on the possible benefit, I recommend wearing blue blockers, especially if you have fair skin and blue or light-colored eyes, if you have any other risk factors, or if you spend lots of time in bright sunlight, or on water, sand, or snow, which reflects sunlight. Alternatively, wear a sun visor when you are outside.

Blue Light and Blue Blockers

Unlike UV light, blue light is visible to us. Blue light waves are what makes the sky, or any object, appear blue. Blue light waves are also very short and scatter easily, so a great deal of the glare we experience from sunlight also comes from blue light. Since we can't see UV light, we also can't see the lens filter used to protect us from UV rays. Conversely, since we can see blue light, we can also see blue blockers, the lens filters that block blue rays. Blue blockers do not act like regular sunglasses. They appear tinted, but they do not reduce overall light or make the world look darker. They alter the appearance of blue and green colors and reduce glare, but they don't affect the way other colors appear. In fact, they may even improve color contrast. Because of these characteristics, blue blockers were very popular a few years ago as sports glasses. Many people with macular degeneration find them particularly helpful regardless of their health benefits because they reduce glare indoors and outdoors while keeping the world bright and visible.

The color that blocks blue is yellow, so blue blockers must contain a yellow tint. Optical shops usually offer a dark, amber lens to provide yellow tint in regular sunglasses. There are ready-made "NOIR" sunglasses that block blue and UV light with a variety of tints, including light yellow, dark yellow, amber, and plum. People with macular degeneration usually prefer dark yellow or plum. NOIR glasses are available as clip-ons and both NOIR and Eschenbach offer large plastic frames that fit over your regular glasses, in the low-vision catalogs listed in the appendix. You can also ask your local optical shop to make you a pair of UV and blue blocker glasses or add blue blockers to your existing glasses. Remember, blue blockers will make your lenses look darker, but they won't make the world look that much darker.

3. Eat a Natural, Low-Fat Balanced Diet with at Least Five Servings per Week of Dark Green Leafy Vegetables

There are many nutrients that function as antioxidants or antioxidant promoters, reducing free radical damage in the body. They include vitamins C and E, selenium, glutathione, and vegetables rich in antioxidants that belong to the carotenoid family. They are usually the brightly colored ones that you are probably already eating: broccoli, carrots, and tomatoes. But you are unlikely to be eating the particular vegetables in the carotenoid family that are rich in lutein and zeaxanthin, two antioxidants important for your macula. That's because these vegetables are less popular and less familiar, particularly outside the South. They are largely the dark green leafy vegetables: kale, collard greens, mustard greens, Swiss chard, spinach, watercress, and parsley. Red peppers and romaine lettuce contain smaller amounts of lutein and zeaxanthin. There have been no studies conclusively showing that eating dark green leafy vegetables prevents or retards macular degeneration. However, it is reasonable to believe there is a link that future studies may confirm. In the meantime, I recommend eating five servings of dark green leafy vegetables per week, averaging 15,000 micrograms of lutein and zeaxanthin per serving (see chart). Because eating a balanced diet is also important, try to vary your intake. The section below entitled "An Eye-Healthy Diet and Vitamins Explained" provides more information on this topic.

Having trouble figuring out how to eat kale or collard greens? You're not alone. Most Americans, especially Northerners and Midwesterners, aren't used to them. To help make dark green leafy vegetables not only healthy but delicious and enjoyable, too, I've asked Seattle chefs Ken and Monica Payson to create a collection of easy high-lutein and zeaxanthin recipes for you. You'll find them in Chapter 4, "Gourmet Greens: Recipes for Your Eyes."

4. Take a Balanced Dose of Vitamins and Minerals

Vitamin supplements are helpful, but don't use them as a crutch for a poor diet. There is simply no true substitute for healthy eating; vitamins can compensate to some degree, but we should always eat well whenever possible. If you take supplements, don't overload on a single vitamin or nutrient. Just as it's not healthy to eat massive amounts of one type of food to the exclusion of others, it's not healthy to take megadoses of anything, or to single out one supplement, say lutein or vitamin E, and take it alone. I recommend taking a balanced multivitamin and mineral supplement that includes the following:

Beta-carotene	20,000–25,000 IU
Lutein	5–10 mg
Vitamin C	500 mg
Vitamin E	400 IU
Zinc	30 mg
Selenium	250 mcg
Copper	2 mg

On many vitamin packages, vitamin A is included in beta-carotene, since some beta-carotene becomes vitamin A in the body. Lutein should also be listed as part of the beta-carotene complex in your vitamins. Do not take beta-carotene by itself, especially if you smoke or drink alcohol regularly. If you smoke, check with your doctor before taking vitamin supplements.

What about the rest of the vitamins in your multivitamin tablets? Amounts of various vitamins and minerals vary from one supplement brand to another. As a rule of thumb, supplements that provide anywhere from the RDA (recommended daily allowance) to two or three times the RDA are optimal. I do not recommend taking megadoses of any vitamin, with the possible exceptions of vitamins E and C since their RDAs are often considered too low. You may also want to look for supplements that have any or all of the following: grape seed extract, gingko biloba, bilberry, taurine, N-acetyl cysteine, and glutathione.

Supplement brands are not standardized or regulated. Different brands use different quality ingredients and different production processes. This is one reason why prices vary so greatly (although the most expensive is not necessarily the best). Vitamin companies often offer anecdotal evidence or customer testimonials to prove their products' value, making comparisons difficult. However, there are good arguments for choosing natural vitamins that are cold processed rather than heat processed, because heat can damage vitamin quality. There are also good arguments for choosing vitamins with vegetable coatings that facilitate dissolution and absorption in the body, rather than synthetic or food varnish coatings. I personally take cold-processed, acqueous coated natural supplements. There are a number of good companies producing food supplements. Consult with your doctor for his or her recommendations.

Keep in mind, however, that all vitamins are processed in one way or another; they have been separated from their original food source and manipulated into tablet form. This means that even if they are from natural sources, they are no longer in exactly the same proportions or forms as they occur in nature. We do not yet know exactly how this impacts the effectiveness of vitamins. Supplements are *supplements*, not *substitutes* for a healthy diet. Above all, supplements are not cure-alls for a junk food diet.

AN EYE-HEALTHY DIET AND VITAMINS EXPLAINED

All vegetables are not created equal. Green beans and cucumbers are low in antioxidants, while kale is off the chart as far as antioxidants for your eyes are concerned. Does that mean you should only eat kale? No, because a balanced diet is the most important priority. To understand how much lutein and zeaxanthin you are getting when you eat various vegetables, check this list:

The Lutein and Zeaxanthin List

VEGETABLE	MICROGRAM OF LUTEIN AND ZEAXANTHIN PER SERVING (3.5 OUNCES)
kale	21,900
collard greens	16,900*
spinach (cooked)	12,600
cress leaf (raw)	12,500*
Swiss chard (raw)	11,000*
parsley (not dried)	10,200
mustard greens	9,400
beet greens	7,700*
okra	6,800*
red pepper	6,800*
romaine lettuce	5,700
broccoli	1,900
peas	1,700
iceberg lettuce	1,400
carrots	260
leaf lettuce	0

*Starred values are imputed by the U.S Department of Agriculture. The remaining values have been laboratory tested.

As you can see, if you eat a Caesar salad with romaine lettuce, you are getting more than four times the amount of lutein and zeaxanthin than you would get if you ate a salad with iceberg lettuce. But eating a spinach salad would give you even more lutein and zeaxanthin than a Caesar salad. Kale, of course, is at the top of the list. One 3.5 ounce serving of kale provides the same amount of lutein and zeaxanthin as fourteen 3.5 ounce servings of iceberg lettuce.

Why Haven't I Heard of Lutein or Zeaxanthin?

Research on nutrition and macular degeneration is very new. It wasn't until 1985 that researchers even knew that lutein and zeaxanthin were important to the macula. The first major study on humans to report that nutrition may play a big role in the development of macular degeneration was the 1994 Eye Disease Case Control Study, conducted by Johanna Seddon, M.D., and her colleagues at Harvard University. The study participants who ate at least five servings a week or more of dark green leafy vegetables, particularly spinach and collard greens, had a 43 percent lower risk of macular degeneration than the participants who ate the smallest amounts of these vegetables, or none at all. In addition to nutrition studies on people, animal studies have been confirming the importance of vitamins and antioxidants to retinal and macular health. In an excellent review of recent research, Max Snodderly, Ph.D., noted new studies showing that monkeys who ate diets deficient in carotenoids for three years had no macular pigment, and monkeys who ate diets deficient in vitamin E for two years developed degeneration of the macula. Although macular degeneration in monkeys is not identical to macular degeneration in humans, these findings are notable. Additionally, guinea pigs who were exposed to high intensity light suffered no eye damage if they were fed vitamin C.

Studies of specific nutrients in humans have produced confusing, conflicting, and sometimes unexpected results. This may be largely because they are designed like prescription drug studies, which typically administer large doses of a single drug to patients and then evaluate the effects. But our bodies are not designed to handle large doses of a single nutrient and, unlike synthetic drugs, the nutrients themselves are not designed to act alone. They rely upon other nutrients to function.

One study, for example, found that smokers who took large doses of beta-carotene had an increased incidence of lung cancer. This news was so disconcerting that it was widely publicized. But smoking seems to reduce the body's capacity to process vitamin A, which may impact its ability to process beta-carotene, and beta-carotene itself cannot function properly without other nutrients.

As a result, this study may not accurately reflect the effects of beta-carotene taken in reasonable amounts and with other nutrients. Clearly, to measure the effects of nutrients in our bodies, we will have to develop research models that can account for this dynamic.

A major nutrition study, part of the AREDS (Age-Related Eye Disease Study), is now underway. It includes several antioxidants, although neither selenium nor lutein. We look forward to the results of AREDS and of future studies that hopefully will take into account all of the nutrients that work as a team in our eyes. In the meantime, it seems clear that lutein, zeaxanthin, and other antioxidants matter to our eyes and to our health; we're just not exactly sure why.

Can I Just Take a Lutein or Zeaxanthin Pill?

Skipping kale and popping a pill may seem appealing, but there's the catch: taking vitamins alone can't fully compensate for a poor diet. Certainly taking lutein alone is unlikely to help. Research suggests that lutein is the most valuable player for our macula's antioxidant team, but lutein, like all vitamins and antioxidants, can't perform alone—it relies on a natural complement of nutrients to be effective. Just taking a lutein pill, or adding spinach to a diet of coffee, steak, and ice cream would be like asking Phil Rizzuto

to field hits from an entire lineup of free radicals all by himself. Vitamins and antioxidants
cannot work alone; neither can any other kind of
nutrient. They always need a team of all the other
players found in a wide variety of fruits and vegetables. We need them all to play ball.

BALANCED DIETS AND THE RDA

During World War II, the government worried
about the possibility of widespread malnutrition.
To assess the public's health, plan for rationing,
and set clear minimum nutrition standards, the
government developed the recommended daily
allowances (RDA). These figures do not represent
an optimal diet, but rather the *minimum* amount
of essential nutrients we need to avoid diseases
and conditions caused or aggravated by deficient
diets. World War II ended without malnutrition
in the United States, but late twentieth century
peacetime malnutrition is a major problem for
Americans.

We eat a lot, but don't eat balanced, varied
diets. We look good, we live a long time, and we
even spend time and money trying to lose weight
and eat less. But we are actually walking around
chronically undernourished in essential vitamins
and minerals. And we've been doing it for at least
twenty years. Indigestion, heartburn, fatigue, fre-

quent colds, allergies, chronic diarrhea, constipation, irritable bowl syndrome, hemorrhoids, high blood pressure, heart disease, some forms of diabetes, some cancers, and very likely macular degeneration are all diet-related conditions. It probably isn't an accident that these are our primary health problems today, and we experience them at near epidemic levels. Certainly diet isn't the whole story: we also have our own genes, live high stress lives, and are exposed to tens of thousands of industrial chemicals. But diet is a big factor, especially when we consider pesticides, food additives, and animal hormones, all of which are common elements of our diet.

In 1978, the USDA conducted a nationwide Food Consumption Survey that contacted 21,500 Americans. Amazingly, not a single American surveyed consumed 100 percent of the RDA for all of the following critical nutrients: vitamins A, B-6, B-12, C, magnesium, calcium, iron, thiamine, and riboflavin. We have become more health-conscious since 1978. The two-martini lunch has disappeared, we know that low-fat diets are important, and you can't smoke on airplanes anymore. But we actually haven't made much progress in terms of consuming adequate amounts of vitamins and minerals. A 1988 USDA survey found that over 70 percent of men and over 80 percent of women failed to get even 66 percent of the RDA for one or more nutrients. In 1990, the Second National Health and

Nutrition Examination Survey revealed that fewer than 10 percent of Americans consumed two servings of fruit and three servings of vegetables a day, 40 percent routinely consumed no fruit or juice, 50 percent consumed no garden vegetable, 70 percent no fruit or vegetable rich in vitamin C, and 80 percent consumed no fruit or vegetable rich in carotenoids. That means that 80 percent of Americans are routinely getting few antioxidants for their maculas, leaving them at higher risk for macular degeneration.

How Do We Wind Up Eating Vitamin-Poor Diets?

While we don't set out trying to avoid nutritious foods, it's incredibly easy to do so. First, we often live fast-paced lives that allow a limited time to choose food and prepare it. With less time, it's harder to be creative; we tend to rely on the same old familiar meals. We also tend to rely on snack foods or packaged foods, like salads in plastic bags or frozen meals, which do not provide adequate nutrition or variety. While many people with macular degeneration have more time to shop, vision loss tends to exacerbate poor nutrition because it makes shopping and cooking more difficult, especially without visual rehabilitation.

Second, we don't realize that we need to eat many more servings of fruit and vegetables than we are accustomed to in order to really meet the

RDA. We usually think of fruit as something we add to pies or cereal. We think of vegetables as side dishes to meat, poultry, or fish. But fruits and vegetables should be our main dishes, while meat, poultry, fish, and starches should be our side dishes. This takes some rethinking of what breakfast, lunch, and dinner should look like.

Third, we don't realize how varied in fruits and vegetables our diets need to be. We often rely on a handful of favorite vegetables that we eat frequently, avoiding all the others or eating them rarely. When we have salads we often return to the same type of lettuce: we always order Caesars, or we always use iceberg lettuce, or we make mixed salads with the same two or three greens every time. When I sat down and assessed my diet a few years ago, I discovered that I regularly ate peas, beans, carrots, and spinach salads, but that was virtually it for vegetables. My diet would've been okay if every vegetable contained every nutrient we need. Eating would then be a matter of quantity rather than variety, but this isn't the case.

Ironically, our vitamin-poor diets may partly be the result of the great availability of food in America. With refrigeration, worldwide shipping, hothouses, and industrialized farms, we can eat almost anything in any season. If spinach and red peppers were only available two months out of the year, we would be excited by their arrival. They might even be our only vegetable options during those two months, and we would eat them in greater quantities. But when vegetables and fruits are available year round, they lose their seasonal appeal and we tend to overlook them, choosing only our favorites month after month.

Finally, medicine has contributed to our poor eating patterns by focusing on pharmaceutical and technological solutions to our health problems while overlooking nutrition. We've been running our cars on poor grade gasoline and oil, and then paying the mechanics to fix the problem. And the mechanics haven't been telling us to take care of our cars, at least not as much as they should. I count myself among those mechanics. I've only started to talk seriously to my patients about nutrition in the last few years. But nutrition is clearly one of the most important things I can talk about, even when it comes to macular degeneration.

EATING A NATURAL, LOW-FAT, RDA-BALANCED DIET

Outlining a complete, natural, low-fat, RDA-balanced diet would take much more room than I have in this book, but I encourage you to use other sources to help create your own. There are many nutrition plans on the market. I recommend using one that emphasizes eating plenty of fruits and vegetables and minimizes chemicals or additives in your diet. My favorite plan is Andrew Weil,

M.D.'s *Eight Weeks to Optimal Healing Power*, which begins with basic alterations in your diet and provides easy-to-follow guidelines. His book is available in print or audiotape. Although it doesn't discuss the RDA of all essential vitamins and minerals, Weil's book does provide a solid, holistic framework from which you can build healthy eating habits and a healthy lifestyle.

At the Very Least, Get the Big Seven

If you decide not to follow a nutrition program or plan, you should at least make sure you are regularly eating foods that give you a natural source of the big seven: beta-carotene, lutein, vitamins C and E, selenium, copper, and zinc. To help you add these foods to your diet, here's a partial list of sources for these nutrients:

NUTRIENT	SOURCES
beta-carotene	red peppers, carrots, avocados, asparagus, squash, sweet potatoes, nectarines, apricots, cantaloupe, mango, papaya, watermelon, kiwi, and dark green leafy vegetables
lutein	kale, collard greens, mustard greens, spinach, parsley, and romaine lettuce

NUTRIENT	SOURCES
vitamin C	red and green peppers, broccoli, Brussels sprouts, turnips, cabbage, citrus fruits, cantaloupe, kiwi, and dark green leafy vegetables
vitamin E	seeds, nuts, whole grains
selenium	wheat germ, oats and bran, fish, egg yolks, chicken, garlic, and red Swiss chard
copper	Brazil nuts, almonds, hazelnuts, walnuts, pecans
zinc	oysters and fish, pumpkin seeds, ginger root, pecans, and Brazil nuts

Use Extra-Virgin Olive Oil and Reduce Saturated Fat

It's important to eat a balanced natural diet that is also low fat. Low-fat diets help prevent high blood pressure and heart disease. You may remember from Chapter 1 that high blood pressure increases your risk of developing wet macular degeneration in your second eye once you show signs of it in your first eye. High blood pressure damages your blood vessels and may contribute to poor circulation and waste management in your eye. Low-fat diets are therefore important for preventing macular degeneration. Low fat means keeping your fat intake to no more than 20 to 30 percent of your total caloric intake. The type of fat you eat, however, makes a big difference.

To eat a truly low-fat diet, you need to reduce saturated fats, because they are hardest on your arteries. Saturated fats are found in meats and dairy products. Although red meat, unskinned chicken, whole milk, butter, and cheese are delicious, the truth is that we were not designed to consume them in large amounts. These foods should not form the core of your diet. Is any fat healthy to eat? Yes, definitely. Our bodies need a certain amount of fat to function. A totally nonfat diet is not healthy either. But some fats are much more healthy for the body than others. The healthiest fat appears to be good quality extra-virgin olive oil. Instead of butter, margarine, vegetable shortening, or other oils, use a good quality extra-virgin olive oil or organic expeller-pressed canola oil, which you can find in health food stores. Always choose cooking methods that minimize fat, like steaming or grilling, rather than pan frying or deep frying.

Avoid Artificial or Treated Foods

Unfortunately, many people try to reduce the amount of saturated fat in their diets by eating commercial fat-free products that use partially hydrogenated vegetable oil or by using polyunsaturated vegetable oils like safflower oil, corn oil, and sunflower oil. There is growing evidence that these oils are not healthy for our bodies, especially when they have been chemically altered or artificially produced. This is a very good reason to choose a good quality extra-virgin olive oil over margarine, which doesn't occur naturally but is made in laboratories by treating vegetable oils with hydrogen.

In fact, I recommend always choosing foods that are as close to nature as possible. Although the additives in our foods, the hormones in our meat, and the pesticides in our vegetables and grains have been approved for use by the government, we still do not understand enough about how the many chemicals we ingest interact with one another and affect our bodies. Better to be safe than sorry. Choose fresh organic fruits, vegetables, and grains over canned fruit, prepackaged salads, and prepackaged baked goods. Choose organic dairy products produced without hormones; labels may say "no hormones," no BGH (Bovine Growth Hormone) or no BHT (Bovine Hormone Treatment). And always try to minimize your consumption of additives, preservatives, artificial colors, flavors, and sweeteners. In general, the shorter the list of ingredients, the better. Some packaged products seem to have more chemicals than food in them. If your grocery store doesn't stock organic produce or dairy products, ask them to.

The more people speak up, the more likely we are to have a choice at the checkout counter. In the meantime, explore your local health food store.

CAN EATING VEGETABLES SLOW MACULAR DEGENERATION?

Researchers do not yet know whether eating green leafy vegetables high in the antioxidants lutein and zeaxanthin can slow the development of macular degeneration once it has begun. Neither do they know for sure that avoiding cigarette smoke will help slow macular degeneration once it has begun. But I advocate both for everyone. I know Chapter 2 delivers some pretty strong warnings about avoiding experimental treatments for macular degeneration until they've been thoroughly studied, so how can I push you to eat vegetables or stop smoking without absolute proof? Because, unlike taking experimental synthetic drugs or having high-risk surgery, eating a healthy diet and avoiding smoke can't hurt you. In fact, we already know that eating a healthy diet and avoiding smoke will improve your overall health. I can't absolutely prove that it will also slow macular degeneration because reliable studies have not yet been conducted, but why wait to find out after the fact?

WHAT ABOUT ZINC?

Zinc is very important for your retina. Many seniors are zinc deficient, which caused researchers to suspect a zinc deficiency at the heart of macular degeneration. In 1988, David Newsome, M.D., of Louisiana State University, and his colleagues conducted a study in which some people were given more than five times the 15 mg RDA of zinc, while others were given a placebo. After a year some of the zinc-treated group experienced vision loss as profound as some members of the placebo group. Dr. Newsome concluded that further studies were needed before high levels of zinc could be recommended for macular degeneration. However, Dr. Newsome's results were reported positively in the media, and many people began taking zinc supplements, sometimes marketed as eye vitamins. In 1996, the Beaver Dam Eye Study concluded that their data weakly supported a positive zinc effect, but they too urged further studies. So the jury is out on zinc, but it certainly doesn't appear to be curative by itself. In the meantime, if we don't know whether or not zinc helps, why not take large doses of zinc just in case? The difficulty with zinc is that large doses can be dangerous. Until we have additional re-search results, I recommend taking twice the RDA, 30 mg, of zinc per day—but do not exceed this amount.

FINALLY, WHAT ABOUT DRINKING WINE?

On a Monday morning last month, a friend of mine called and requested a prescription for red wine. "I just read in the papers that red wine helps with macular degeneration," he quipped. "Maybe with a prescription my insurance will cover a few bottles of Bordeaux!" By the late afternoon, my office phones were ringing off their hooks. Could red wine really make a difference? Everyone wanted to know. The study that raised the question was conducted by Thomas O. Obisesan, M.D., at Howard University. Dr. Obisesan gave 3,072 adults questionnaires and found that 9 percent of the nondrinkers had macular degeneration, while only 4 percent of the wine drinkers did. The beer and liquor drinkers ended up halfway between these two groups. It may be that the antioxidant phytoalexin resvertrol, which is found in red wine, helps. It would be nice if we could add red wine to a kale salad for the perfect eye-healthy dinner, but the research on wine and ARMD is still inconclusive. In the meantime, we do know that it is not the alcohol content in red wine that makes a difference. The Beaver Dam Eye Study actually reported an increase in macular degeneration among beer drinkers. And an Australian study found no connection between macular degeneration and alcohol consumption.

CHAPTER 4

Gourmet Greens:
Recipes for Your Eyes

You probably already eat spinach, red peppers, and romaine lettuce. But unless you're a Southerner, the dark green leafy vegetables that are rich in antioxidants for your maculas aren't likely to be familiar. Many people admit they wouldn't recognize kale if it were walking down the street, much less know what to do with it in the kitchen. My father, who has macular degeneration, set out to eat more kale but complained that kale stalks were awfully stringy and tough when you ate them raw. "Kale stalks?" I asked. "Yes," he replied. "Kale doesn't seem to have much in the way of leaves, so I eat the stalks." I imagined a typical kale bunch with long, thick, bluish-green leaves. "Look!" my father exclaimed, taking a big bag of fresh parsley out of the refrigerator. "Well," I said, "parsley's good for you, too."

Even if you can pick kale out of a crowd, you may still have a creeping suspicion that it would taste rather unsavory. Despite Popeye, dark green leafy vegetables have never had the same appeal as a fine steak. The good news, though, is that dark greens are actually exceptionally easy to embrace. Unlike many other vegetables, most dark greens have a mild flavor that blends well into sandwiches, salads, soups, and pastas. You can add them to your own cooking without changing the flavors you love. And dark greens can be delicious on their own, too. To encourage my own family to eat more dark greens, I asked Seattle chefs Ken and Monica Payson to develop a collection of original gourmet greens recipes. You'll find them here, along with a few simple family favorites. My father loves them all, and I hope you'll enjoy them, too. Bon appetit!

Low Vision and Gourmet Greens

The recipes in this chapter are for everyone. Good nutrition is prevention, and cooking is fun. Share these recipes with your family and friends of all ages. If you have low vision, the easiest way to add dark greens to your diet is to use the suggestions below for adding them to familiar recipes for main dishes, soups, sandwiches, and salads. You can also cook them separately using the Simple Greens recipes below. Most of the gourmet recipes in this chapter are easy, although some call for a number of spices, which makes their ingredient lists look long. If you or your friend or family member has low vision, take this chapter to a photocopy shop and have it enlarged to a print size you can easily read. Collect them with your other large print recipes in a handy binder. Chapter 13, Saving Sight in Your Home, has cooking and magnifier tips for the kitchen that you may find helpful.

Using Dark Greens in Your Cooking

Dark greens are generally mild and blend well with other foods, especially when cooked. Of them all, mustard greens have the biggest personality. They take their name from their strong, almost horseradishy bite. Use them in place of fresh lettuce to add zip to salads and sandwiches. Spinach is a bit earthy, collards are slightly sour, and Swiss chard sometimes has a beety flavor. Kale is one of the gentlest greens and will go with many recipes. You can also heat dark greens separately as a side dish, using the Simple Greens recipes below, or eat them raw.

You can interchange any of the greens in this chapter's recipes. If you dislike chard or can't find kale at the supermarket, you can always use spinach or mustard greens instead, and vice versa. Fresh, healthy greens should not have a strong odor, unless they are overcooked. If you notice a strong odor, your greens may not be fresh or you may be cooking them for too long.

EYE-HEALTHY DARK GREENS AND VEGETABLES

kale	beet greens
Swiss chard	spinach
cress leaf	parsley
okra	red pepper
collard greens	romaine lettuce
mustard greens	

Adding Dark Greens to Your Menu

- Toss mustard greens and spinach into your regular salads.

- Choose Caesar or spinach salads over iceberg lettuce salads.

- Substitute mustard greens and spinach for lettuce in almost any sandwich.

- Add red pepper to spaghetti sauce, sandwiches, and salads.

- Add Swiss chard stems to your favorite soups or chowders.

- Add a handful of chopped kale or mustard greens to scrambled eggs or an omelet.

- Add a cup or two of dark greens to your favorite casserole before baking.

Buying and Storing Dark Greens

All greens are, well, green, with slight variations in hue. You can distinguish among them in the grocery by the store tags or by their appearance and feel. Both kale and mustard greens have long ruffled leaves. Mustard greens are a bright, springy green, while kale has a bluish tinge and a slightly stiff, waxy feel. Swiss chard has red veins and stalks, oval shaped leaves, and a crinkly texture. Collard greens have almost white veins and stalks, and large round leaves that are a bit stiff. Spinach, of course, is dark green and has spear shaped, smooth leaves. When choosing your greens, select bunches that are firm. Leathery, wilted, yellow leaf edges or a strong smell are sure signs that the bunch has been sitting for too long.

Fresh greens will store well in the refrigerator for a few days. You might find it easier to wash and trim your greens all at once and then store them in the refrigerator until you need them. Greens grow in loose, open bunches, so they collect a lot of dirt. Be sure to rinse them well on both sides, or soak them in a sink full of cold water. Dry them in an inexpensive plastic salad spinner or place them in a colander to drain. If you do wash them before storing, be sure to dry the leaves thoroughly or they won't keep. Greens store well in regular plastic produce bags with a strip of paper towel at the bottom of the bag to absorb extra moisture. Or you can buy Ziploc perforated vegetable storage bags that do all the work for you. In either case, be sure to press out excess air before sealing.

While fresh vegetables are always best, you might find it more convenient to use frozen greens. They are available in the frozen vegetable section of most supermarkets. Keep in mind, though, that frozen greens sometimes have a stronger flavor than fresh ones. Be sure to thaw and drain frozen greens by squeezing out the excess water before adding to recipes.

Measuring Greens

Cooking vegetables is unlike baking pastries because precisely measuring the main ingredient—the vegetable—is not critical to the outcome, as measuring the flour would be in baking a cake. Greens are sold in bunches or sometimes, as in the case of spinach, in bags. There may be some variation in the precise weight from one bunch to another, but the difference will not be significant to the recipe. Many of the recipes call for a "bunch" of greens. A bunch is whatever your market sells as a bunch!

SIMPLE GREENS . . .
AND GOURMET GREENS:
RECIPES FOR YOUR EYES

Simple Greens

Easy Kale
1 pound mustard greens or kale
your favorite spices

Remove stems of mustard greens or kale. Wash thoroughly and boil in 1 inch of water in covered pot for 5 to 10 minutes, or microwave. Add any one or several of the following spices: oregano, garlic, onion, lemon or lime juice, wine vinegar, or nutmeg to taste. Our favorite is nutmeg.

Easy Swiss Chard
1 bunch Swiss chard
extra-virgin olive oil or canola oil
basil, nutmeg, or oregano

Chop leaves and slice stems crosswise. Put 1 tablespoon of oil in pan and heat 1 minute. Add 1 tablespoon water and the greens. Cover and cook 2 minutes. Add your choice of: basil, nutmeg, or oregano to taste.

Baked Spinach
2 10-ounce packages frozen chopped spinach,
defrosted and drained

3 cups low-fat cottage cheese
1 cup plain bread crumbs
⅔ cup grated Parmesan cheese
1 egg white
4 whole eggs
extra-virgin olive or canola oil
nutmeg

Preheat the oven to 350 degrees. Put well-drained spinach in large bowl. Add cottage cheese. Add grated cheese and ¾ cup of the bread crumbs. Beat 2 whole eggs and the egg white in a separate bowl. Add to spinach-cheese mixture and mix well. Spread oil lightly on 9-inch square baking pan, add ¼ cup bread crumbs. Bake for 5 minutes to brown the crumbs. Spread the spinach mixture over the crumbs. Beat the other 2 eggs and pour over the mixture in pan. Sprinkle top lightly with nutmeg. Bake 45 minutes. Cool for 10 minutes and cut in 3-inch squares. This recipe can be doubled and frozen. You can freeze squares individually for single portions.

Great Greens 'n' Garlic
1 pound kale or collard greens
¼ cup olive oil
¼ cup garlic, peeled and thinly sliced
½ teaspoon red-pepper flakes
salt
freshly ground black pepper
lemon wedges

Wash greens, cut stems into 1-inch pieces, and chop leaves coarsely. Leave greens wet. In large saucepan put olive oil, garlic, pepper flakes, salt, and pepper. Cook over medium heat for 1 minute. Add greens to saucepan and cover. Cook over medium-high heat for 5 minutes. Greens should still be a little firm. Uncover and continue cooking and stirring over medium heat until liquid is almost gone and greens are tender. Don't overcook. Serve with lemon. Goes very well with fish.

Gourmet Greens

BY KEN AND MONICA PAYSON

SALADS

Spinach Salad with Orange Sesame Vinaigrette

Many people go through their lives thinking of salad as little more than background. But the best salads make your mouth tingle. Orange and onion are a pair made in heaven and a little bit of sesame brings all the flavors together while adding a little crunch. Be sure to use toasted sesame oil or you will miss all that warm, nutty flavor.

2 tablespoons apple cider vinegar
1½ teaspoons soy sauce
2 tablespoons canola oil

1 tablespoon toasted sesame oil
¼ teaspoon black pepper
1 small can mandarin orange segments,
   drained
8 cups fresh spinach, torn
½ cup thinly sliced red onion
1 teaspoon toasted sesame seeds

Whisk together the vinegar, soy sauce, canola oil, sesame oil, and black pepper in a salad bowl. Add the mandarin orange segments, spinach, and onions. Toss well. Garnish with sesame seeds.
   Serves 4.

Oshitashi (Japanese Spinach Salad)

   The Japanese typically build their meals around rice, adding small dishes of meat, pickles, and vegetables as an accompaniment. Oshitashi is delicious with hot rice for lunch. If that seems a bit too exotic, try it as side salad with fish or chicken.

2 bunches fresh spinach, washed with stems
   intact
2 tablespoons sesame seeds
2 tablespoons soy sauce
2 teaspoons sugar

Heat a small pan over medium heat. Add the sesame seeds and toast until light brown and aromatic, about 5 minutes. Transfer the sesame seeds to a small bowl to cool. Boil water in a pot large enough to comfortably fit both bunches of spinach. Blanch the spinach for 30 seconds. Immediately plunge the spinach into a bowl of ice water to stop the cooking process. While the spinach cools, coarsely grind the sesame seeds in a *scrupulously clean* spice grinder or with a mortar and pestle. Grind for only a few seconds so the sesame seeds are the texture of corn meal. Do not make a paste! Mix the sesame seeds, soy sauce, and sugar in a salad bowl. Remove the spinach from the water and squeeze out the excess water. Chop coarsely and add to the soy sauce mixture. Mix well and serve at room temperature.

Serves 4.

Romaine Salad with Red Peppers, Toasted Walnuts, and Goat Cheese

This salad makes a simple lunch with bread. Have a ripe pear for dessert to complement the flavors. Or serve it alongside simple spaghetti in marinara sauce at dinner. If the flavor of goat cheese is too pungent for you, any creamy, crumbly cheese will do.

DRESSING

½ shallot, finely minced*

*If you do not have a shallot, substitute 1 tablespoon finely minced yellow or red onion. But keep in mind that the flavor will be much stronger.

1½ tablespoons orange juice (fresh squeezed
 is best but bottled is okay)
1 tablespoon champagne or apple cider
 vinegar
¼ teaspoon salt
freshly ground black pepper to taste
2 tablespoons olive oil

Mix the shallot, orange juice, vinegar, salt, and
pepper. Whisk in the oil until all ingredients are
well combined. Set aside so the flavors can blend
while you prepare the salad. You may need to whisk
the dressing again before pouring over the salad.

SALAD

½ cup walnut pieces
1 small head romaine lettuce
1 small red pepper, seeded and thinly sliced
2 ounces goat cheese (about a 1-by-2-inch
 chunk)

Preheat oven to 350 degrees. Spread the walnuts
out in a pie pan and toast in the oven for 10 minutes. Remove from the oven and set aside to cool.
Wash and dry the romaine leaves and tear them
into medium size pieces (about 1 to 2 inches).
Place the lettuce in a large bowl. You should have
about 4 to 6 cups of lettuce. Crumble the goat
cheese into the lettuce. Add the sliced red pepper.
If necessary, cut the walnuts into approximately

pea-size chunks and add to the bowl. Pour the dressing over the salad and toss well.

Serves 4.

SOUPS

Portuguese Kale Soup

This is a thick, hearty soup, perfect for a cold day. If you can find it, turkey sausage is a healthy alternative to beef or pork. Serve with bread and salad for a light but satisfying dinner or lunch.

2 tablespoons olive oil
½ pound chorizo or Italian sausage
1 medium onion, chopped
3 cloves garlic, minced
2 stalks celery, chopped
6 cups water
4 cups kale, chopped
salt
black pepper

Remove the sausage from its casing. Heat a soup pot over medium heat. Add the olive oil. When the oil is hot, add the sausage and cook until lightly browned, about 4 minutes. Add the onion and garlic. Cook until translucent, about 4 minutes. Add the celery and cook 3 more minutes. Add the water and kale and bring to a boil. Reduce the heat to a simmer and cook, partially covered, for 1 hour. Add salt and black pepper to taste.

Serves 4.

Lentil Soup with Mustard Greens

This is one of our favorite soups, a real standby. If you want to cut out the fat or you don't have time to sauté all the vegetables, simply add everything to the soup pot with the stock and simmer until thick and creamy. Be sure not to add the salt until the lentils are fully cooked or they will be tough. Serve with bread and salad, or over rice.

2 tablespoons olive oil
1 onion, chopped
2 cloves garlic, minced
1 stalk celery, chopped
1 carrot, chopped
1 teaspoon ground cumin
1 teaspoon ground coriander
1 teaspoon oregano
¼ teaspoon allspice
6 cups mustard greens
1½ cups lentils
8 cups chicken stock
salt
black pepper

Heat 2 tablespoons olive oil in a large saucepan over medium-high heat. Add the onion and garlic. Cook until soft, about 3 minutes. Add the celery, carrot, cumin, coriander, oregano, and allspice. Cook for another 3 minutes. Add the mustard greens, lentils, and chicken stock. Bring to a boil. Reduce heat to a simmer and cook, covered, for 45 minutes. Add salt and black pepper to taste.

Serves 6.

Many Greens Soup

A smooth deep green, this soup is a little more elegant than the previous two. Add croutons for a satisfying lunch, or serve for dinner with roasted red pepper and smoked mozzarella sandwiches.

1 tablespoon olive oil
1 large yellow onion, finely chopped
4 garlic cloves, minced or pressed
1 large potato, peeled and diced
2 large carrots, peeled and diced
¼ cup white wine
1 bunch kale, stems removed and leaves
    shredded
1 bunch chard, stems removed and leaves
    shredded
1 bunch spinach, stems removed and leaves
    shredded
3½ cups chicken stock*

*To make a bisque, substitute one cup of milk for one cup of stock. Add the milk at the very end after you have pureed the soup, and be very careful not to boil.

1½ teaspoons salt
freshly ground black pepper
grated Parmesan cheese

Heat the olive oil in a medium soup pot. Add the onions, ½ teaspoon salt, and a few grinds of pepper to taste. Sauté over medium heat until the onions are soft, about 5 to 7 minutes. Add the garlic, potatoes, and carrots. Sauté until the vegetables are heated through, about 5 minutes. Add ½ cup stock, cover the pot, and cook for 10 minutes. When the vegetables are tender, add the wine and simmer until nearly all the liquid evaporates, about 1 to 2 minutes. Stir in the kale, chard, 1 teaspoon salt, and 3 cups of stock. Cover pot and simmer for 10 to 15 minutes. Add the spinach and cook for another 3 to 5 minutes until the spinach is just wilted. Puree the soup in a blender until it is very smooth. Keep in mind that the hot liquid will expand in the blender so puree in several batches. (A hand blender will also work for this but will not handle the more fibrous kale as well as a traditional blender, and your soup will not be as smooth.) Return to the soup pot and thin with a little more stock or water if the soup seems too thick. Heat over low heat until just hot. Serve immediately, sprinkled with Parmesan cheese.

Cajun Collard Greens

Collard greens are classic Southern fare. The versatile seasonings in this dish make it an easy accompaniment for any meat or bean dish. Or try it with our Gumbo (recipe below).

2 tablespoons canola oil
1 medium onion, diced
2 cloves garlic, minced
½ teaspoon basil
½ teaspoon thyme
¼ teaspoon cumin
½ teaspoon black pepper
1 16-ounce package frozen collard greens
½ cup chicken stock
1 tablespoon Tabasco
salt

Heat vegetable oil in a 10-inch skillet over medium-high heat. Add onion, garlic, basil, thyme, cumin, and black pepper. Cook for 3 to 4 minutes until onion begins to brown. Add collard greens and chicken stock. Cover, reduce heat to medium, and cook for 20 minutes. Add Tabasco and salt to taste.

Serves 4.

MAIN DISHES

Roasted Peppers, Spinach, and Smoked Mozzarella Sandwich

A combination that goes well beyond the common, this sandwich makes an easy lunch or dinner without being boring. If you don't feel like adventuring into new territory right away, try a good old-fashioned turkey sandwich with mustard greens instead of lettuce.

    1 16-ounce baguette
    1 clove garlic, halved
    2 tablespoons olive oil
    1 6-ounce jar roasted red peppers, drained
    8 ounces smoked mozzarella, thinly sliced
    2 cups packed fresh spinach, cut into ½-inch
        ribbons
    1 tablespoon red wine vinegar

Position rack in the upper third of the oven and preheat the broiler. Cut the baguette in half lengthwise and rub with the cut side of the garlic. Drizzle olive oil over both halves, place on foil-lined baking sheet, and toast lightly under the broiler, about 30 seconds. Distribute the red peppers evenly over one side of the baguette. Distribute the cheese over the other side of the baguette. Broil until the cheese begins to brown, 1 to 2 minutes. Arrange the spinach on the bottom half of the baguette and sprinkle with the vinegar. Place other half on top and cut into 4 pieces.

Serves 4.

Ham and Kale Casserole

We love this casserole because it tastes and feels like classic American fare—creamy, smooth, and comforting. Like most of the recipes in this chapter, this casserole makes a simple lunch or dinner with just a salad on the side.

> 1 bunch kale, finely chopped
> 2 tablespoons butter
> 1 medium onion, chopped
> 1 cup mushrooms, sliced
> ½ teaspoon salt
> 2 tablespoons flour
> 1½ cups low-fat milk
> 2 cups diced ham
> 2 cups cooked rice
> 1 cup grated cheddar or Swiss cheese

Preheat oven to 350 degrees. Blanch the kale in boiling water for 2 minutes. Drain and set aside. Melt 2 tablespoons of the butter in a small saucepan over medium heat. Add the onion and cook for 3 minutes, until translucent. Add the mushrooms and cook for 4 minutes more. Add the flour and salt. Cook for 2 minutes, stirring occasionally. Adjust the heat if necessary to prevent the flour from browning. Slowly add the milk while stirring with a whisk. Continue stirring and cook until thickened, 3 to 4 minutes. Remove from heat. In a large mixing bowl combine milk mixture, ham, rice, cheese, and cooked kale. Pour into 2½ quart casserole and smooth the top with a spatula. Cook uncovered for 45 minutes until browned on top.

Serves 4.

New Orleans Gumbo

Gumbo is a traditional Louisiana stew with rice. Hearty and a bit spicy, it's a meal in itself. A simple salad of fresh romaine lightens things up a bit. Or for a real Southern meal, serve with Cajun Collard Greens on the side. (Recipe above.)

  2 tablespoons canola oil
  2 tablespoons butter
  2 cups onions, chopped
  4 garlic cloves, minced
  4 cups okra, sliced
  2 cups red bell pepper, chopped
  3 teaspoons paprika
  1 teaspoon black pepper
  ½ teaspoon thyme
  ½ teaspoon sage
  ½ pound kielbasa, sliced
  6 cups chicken stock
  1 teaspoon salt
  ½ pound small shrimp, peeled
  1 tablespoon Tabasco
  cooked rice
  ½ cup green onions, chopped

Heat the oil and butter over medium-high heat in large saucepan. Add the onions and garlic and cook until lightly brown, about 5 minutes. Add the okra and cook, stirring occasionally, another 10 minutes. Add the red bell pepper, paprika, black pepper, thyme, sage, kielbasa, chicken stock, and salt and bring to boil. Reduce heat to low and cook covered for 1 hour. Add the shrimp and Tabasco and cook another 2 minutes. Serve over hot rice and garnish with green onions.

Serves 4.

Angel Hair Pasta with Chicken, Spinach, and Olives

Pasta is a staple in our house because it's cheap, easy, delicious, and filling. This recipe should give you a good sense of how versatile both pasta and greens are. A natural pair when you need to throw together a quick meal!

1 pound dried angel hair pasta
4 tablespoons olive oil
4 cloves garlic, minced
4 anchovy fillets, minced
1 pound boneless skinless chicken breast, sliced into $\frac{1}{4}$-by-1-inch pieces
1 6-ounce can ripe black olives, coarsely chopped
$\frac{1}{2}$ cup chicken stock

6 cups fresh spinach, shredded
2 tablespoons lemon juice
salt
grated Parmesan

Bring 4 quarts of water to a boil with 1 tablespoon salt. Cover and keep at a slow boil until you are ready to cook the pasta. Meanwhile, heat the olive oil in a large nonstick pan over medium-high heat. Add the garlic and anchovy and cook for 30 seconds. Add the chicken and cook, stirring occasionally until the chicken surface is uniformly white, about 3 minutes. Add the olives and chicken stock and reduce heat to low. Cook the pasta according to the instructions on the package. Add the pasta, spinach, and lemon juice to the pan and toss until combined. Add salt to taste. Garnish with Parmesan.

Serves 4.

Chicago-Style Spinach and Mushroom Pizza

Pizza isn't everyday fare, but it's nice to have a great recipe when you feel like being adventurous and when you want to be rewarded for your efforts. Chicago style stuffed pizza can't be beat for good looks or flavor. Among cheeses, mozzarella is already relatively low in fat. For even less fat without sacrificing taste, use skim or low-fat mozzarella.

CRUST

1½ teaspoons sugar
1¼ cups warm water
1 package active dried yeast
¼ cup cornmeal
2 teaspoons salt
¼ cup olive oil
4 to 5 cups flour

FILLING

2 tablespoons olive oil
1 medium onion, chopped
½ pound mushrooms, sliced
1 10-ounce package frozen spinach, thawed
      and squeezed dry
½ pound grated mozzarella cheese
1 16-ounce can diced tomatoes, drained
1 teaspoon oregano
½ teaspoon basil
½ teaspoon sugar
¼ teaspoon salt
¼ teaspoon black pepper
2 tablespoons grated Parmesan

PREPARING THE CRUST

In a mixing bowl, dissolve the sugar in water and sprinkle the yeast on top. After 5 minutes add the cornmeal, salt, and olive oil. Stir, adding flour, until the dough is shaggy and too thick to stir.

Scrape onto a floured surface and knead, adding flour until the dough no longer sticks. Continue kneading until the dough is the consistency of an earlobe, about 10 minutes. Place the dough in an oiled bowl and cover with plastic wrap. Let rise until doubled in bulk, about 2 hours.

PREPARING THE FILLING

Heat the remaining 2 tablespoons olive oil in a large skillet over medium-high heat. Add the onion and ¼ teaspoon salt, and cook until soft, about 3 minutes. Add the mushrooms and cook another 3 minutes.

ASSEMBLING THE PIZZA

Preheat oven to 400 degrees. Punch down the risen dough. Remove it from the bowl and knead lightly until smooth. Divide the dough in half and press out one portion into a 12-inch pan until it reaches one inch up the sides. Spread the cheese evenly over the dough. Spread the onions, mushrooms, and spinach over the cheese. Roll out the remaining dough and cover the filling, pressing the edges of the two layers of dough together. Combine the tomatoes, oregano, basil, remaining ¼ teaspoon of salt, and black pepper. Spread tomato mixture evenly over the surface of the pizza. Sprinkle with the Parmesan and bake for 30 minutes.

Serves 4.

Joe's Special

Joe's Special is essentially fancy scrambled eggs. It's perfect for brunch, lunch, or dinner. Serve with bread or toast and salad for a simple, homey meal.

3 eggs
¼ teaspoon Tabasco
2 tablespoons canola oil
¼ cup chopped red onions
½ teaspoon minced garlic
6 ounces lean ground beef*
2 cups sliced mushrooms
½ teaspoon salt
2 packed cups fresh spinach, shredded
¼ teaspoon pepper

Beat the eggs with the Tabasco until well combined and set aside. Heat a 10-inch nonstick sauté pan over medium-high heat. Add the oil and swirl to coat the bottom of the pan. Add the onions and garlic. Cook for 3 minutes until translucent. Add the ground beef and cook until no longer pink, about 3 minutes. Add the mushrooms and salt. Cook for 4 minutes until the mushrooms are soft. Add the spinach and toss until the spinach wilts, about 30 seconds. Add the eggs and stir occasionally until the eggs are set.

Serves 2.

*Lean ground turkey also works well for this recipe.

PART II:

Experiencing ARMD

CHAPTER 5

I Am Not Blind: The Shock of ARMD

I am not blind. Do not tell me that I am blind. I refuse to be blind. I hate that word.

—Grace Olsen

When I first met Grace Olsen, she was wearing a blue wool dress with pearl buttons. She had her hair in a pretty blond bob, and she held her chin up. At eighty-two, she looked not a day over seventy, and she was fierce. She eyed me unapologetically and observed that she'd been to two other ophthalmologists since she'd been diagnosed with macular degeneration, including her retinal specialist, and none of them had much to say. "My son thinks I should go to the School for the Blind in Kalamazoo," she said evenly, "but I am not blind. Do not tell me that I am blind. I refuse to be blind. I hate that word." No, I agreed, she was not blind and she would not go blind from macular degeneration. But with 20/200 acuity in both eyes, she did have low vision. "You have no idea what this is like," Grace continued, her voice becoming softer. "It's such a shock. You cannot understand unless it happens to you." And then she quietly began to cry.

YOU HAVE NO IDEA WHAT THIS IS LIKE

Grace was right. I have no idea what it's like to have macular degeneration. I am already sixty, though, my father has advanced macular degeneration, and I have his light blue eyes. Since those are all risk factors, I may know in a few years. But talking right now with Grace, I could not tell her that I really understood. Listening and imagining are not the same as living. This is one of the toughest things facing anyone with macular degeneration. It's an experience that's hard to convey. It's not even a condition that's widely known.

Macular What? or The Macarena

"Macular what?" people often say, as Zelda Grant did when she was diagnosed. "I had never heard of macular degeneration before. Suddenly I found myself having to explain it to everyone. When I saw stiff Al Gore do that silly Macarena dance at the 1996 Democratic Convention, I started calling it the Macarena. Now people say, 'The Macarena what?' "

Although macular degeneration is receiving

more public attention, I had to agree with Zelda when she pointed out how amazing it is that more than 1.5 million Americans have sight loss from a condition that few seem to understand. Macular degeneration causes more vision loss than glaucoma, cataracts, and diabetic retinopathy combined. It is the number one cause of vision loss in the United States and Europe, and seniors are its number one targets. "It's hard to have something that changes your whole life, and no one's heard of it," Zelda observed dryly. "I do chuckle to myself when someone marvels at how they named a vision problem after a line dance. Yep, I say. You'd be surprised at the things they do these days."

It's Hard to See if It Isn't Happening to You

We usually associate vision loss with looking different. We expect people with vision loss to be blind, and blind people to have obviously damaged or unfocused eyes. But if you have macular degeneration, you won't look any different to your neighbors, friends, or family. You make proper eye contact with people, just like you always have, so they are unlikely to realize that you can't see them clearly. In familiar surroundings, you probably don't appear to be any less competent or confident than you did ten years ago. You may also be able to do much of what you did before macular degeneration, although it may take two or three times longer. "I used to be able to change a doorknob in ten minutes," Joe Toscano reported. "Now I can still do it, but it takes over an hour. An hour for a doorknob! I'm always worried about how much worse it will get. But the neighbors have no idea. To them I look and act just like the same old Joe."

Because you look and act so much like you always have, even best friends and spouses may find it difficult to remember what you can and can't see. "It's amazing how easily even the people closest to me forget," Dolly Kowalski told me. "My friend Maria and I have dinner together almost every night. Last week we went out to an Italian restaurant and Maria says in a disappointed voice, 'Dolly, you haven't said anything about my new necklace.' I just said, 'Have you lost your mind? I can't see that necklace! I didn't even know you were wearing one!' Maria was very quiet. So I said, 'Pass the dates, please.' Then she said gently, 'They're not dates, Dolly, they're olives.' So I winked at her. I figured they were olives. But honestly! She knows I can't recognize people when they walk into the room. What in the world would possess her to think I could see a little pearl necklace?"

SO WHAT CAN YOU SEE?

To say you have macular degeneration is to say that your central vision is affected, but it doesn't say *how much* it is affected. You may have 20/40 visual acuity or 20/600 or anything in between (see Chapter 1 for an explanation of visual acuity measurements).

To say you have macular degeneration also doesn't say *how* your vision is affected. And *how* turns out to matter a great deal. ARMD reduces central vision, but it also affects contrast sensitivity, glare sensitivity, and depth perception. All of these factors influence your overall experience of seeing.

It's helpful to understand these factors and be aware of what you can and can't see. It's also very helpful for your friends and family to understand your experience of seeing. But remember that to say that you have macular degeneration, or to say you have a certain visual acuity, doesn't say much about what you can or can't do with your vision. It's true that if you have 20/200 vision you aren't likely to qualify for a driver's license. But driver's licenses are legally regulated according to visual acuity. Most activities in life are not. Don't make the leap between being aware of your vision and labeling yourself with limitations.

Contrast Sensitivity

Low contrast sensitivity explains much of what seems peculiar about vision affected by ARMD. For example, most people find it difficult to understand or explain why they can see a two-inch letter in a newspaper headline, but they can't recognize their own grandchildren's faces. Most of their relatives find this confusing, too. Maria fell right into this divide when she went to dinner with Dolly and fished for a compliment on the necklace. Dolly could see the olives on the table, after all, so why couldn't she see Maria's necklace?

The answer is that Dolly has low contrast sensitivity. Macular degeneration may decrease contrast sensitivity because it affects the ability of the rod and cone cells to tell similar colors or shades apart. As a result, many people with macular degeneration find it difficult to distinguish between navy blue and brown, or pastel pink and pastel orange. In fact, any object that isn't in sharp contrast to its background may be difficult to see. Black-white contrast combinations are always the best. That's why Dolly can see black olives on a white plate; they have excellent contrast and are therefore much easier to see than a pearl necklace against a white sweater, regardless of the size of the necklace.

Human faces are the worst. They have terrible contrast. No matter what color your skin may be, it's probably all the same color, so the contours of your features blend together. "I have four beautiful little grandchildren," Dolly Kowalski said. "They all look equally beautiful to me. In fact, they all look the same. I call their visits playing the Who's Kissing Me Now? game. My daughter says, 'How can they look alike? They have such different features.' But what's a nose or a chin when it's the same color as a forehead?" If we all had either extremely light or extremely dark skin, neon orange eyes and lips, and a contrasting-color nose, we'd be much more visible. Until that happens, macular degeneration may make it easier to see a two-inch-high black letter standing against white paper than to see a grandchild's nose. "They're all my favorites," Dolly said. "I tell them, 'Grandma can't see your pretty smiles so you have to laugh out loud when you're happy.' So they fall over themselves guffawing. My daughter always comes running in and tries to quiet the ruckus."

Glare Sensitivity

Glare sensitivity also affects many people with macular degeneration. Joe Toscano's experience is typical. "I'm actually not too bothered by contrast, especially since Inez matches up my clothes," Joe said, flipping a fluorescent light switch in his kitchen. "But look! I can hardly open my eyes with this glare. When I'm in someone else's house, I find it difficult to see as much as I usually can if they have fluorescent lighting or if the room is flooded with sunlight. I carry a pair of light yellow NOIR sunglasses to cut the glare indoors. My old friend Tony says to me, 'Hey Joe! What are you doing wearing those goggles inside?' I say, 'Hey, Tony, do you want to play cards or not? No goggles, no cards. You should wear them, too, they'd make you look better.' Tony just smiles. We've been giving each other a hard time for seventy years. We met in grade school. How about that?"

Depth Perception

Buddy Burmester doesn't notice glare as much as Joe, but he does have poor depth perception. Poor depth perception may occur when one eye is more affected by ARMD than the other, throwing the two out of sync. It may also result from low contrast sensitivity. Contrast sensitivity enhances our depth perception because we use variations in shades and sharp lines to perceive three-dimensional objects. "Have you ever seen a coin at the bottom of a pool, dived for it, and found that it's not where you expected it to be? That's macular degeneration for me," Buddy Burmester said. "It's like living with permanent pool vision. I can't tell you how many times I've reached for a soda can and it's not exactly where I think it is. It's such a difficult experience to convey to anyone else. It's just a difficult experience, period. I'm not even used to it yet."

One of the most frustrating consequences of poor depth perception is that it may make walking in unfamiliar places more precarious. Since walking is important for transportation and exercise, if you have poor depth perception consider using a walking cane for stability or walk with a friend. Explore other forms of physical activity and exercise, like riding a stationary bicycle, swimming, pool running, weight lifting, gentle stretching classes, or relaxation yoga. Above all, try not to let poor depth perception contribute to isolation and lower activity levels.

THE SHOCK OF DISCOVERING ARMD

For some people, macular degeneration comes on gradually, as it did for Sam Weinberg, whose dry ARMD progressed very slowly for fifteen years. For others, like Zelda Grant, macular degeneration comes in waves. Initially Zelda was diagnosed with dry macular degeneration, but she experienced only minor vision loss in one eye. Three years later, Zelda was at a local conference. As she looked over the presentation schedule posted on a board in the lobby, she reached up and rubbed one eye. To Zelda's shock, the presentation schedule disappeared. She went immediately to her doctor and discovered that she had developed wet macular degeneration. Like Zelda, Grace Olsen also experienced macular degeneration as a sudden, unexpected shock.

Shock Is Not Just Surprise

Feeling shocked can be traumatic itself, above and beyond the actual life change or loss we sustain from the event that shocked us. When we are shocked by a sudden life-threatening or life-changing event, we are more than surprised by something negative. We are hit with a feeling of powerlessness to stop what is happening to us. To a large degree, our sense of security in the world is predicated on our faith that we can determine our present and our future, and that we have options. Of course, we can and we do. But shock throws that faith into question. Feeling shocked without hearing about options and paths for action can exacerbate both the shock and the original problem, eventually contributing to depression. To counter shock, it's very important to seek support and visual rehabilitation as soon as you find out about your condition. Unfortunately, many people who have macular degeneration weren't told about resources and rehabilitation programs in their area. They may have received little attention when they were diagnosed. This was Grace Olsen's experience. If this was your experience, too, it's never too late. Seek support now. Like Grace you may still have residual feelings of shock. You may wonder why it happened the way it did.

GRACE OLSEN'S STORY

It happened in the summer of 1997. In June, I bought a beautiful gray Lincoln my husband would have loved. It reminded me so much of him. I drove myself up to Traverse City for the Fourth of July. The humidity was terrible. And the road signs seemed so far away, as if I were looking at them through smoke. I thought it was the heat—waves of hot air rising from the cement. I remember singing, "Fly Me to the Moon" and squinting at the road signs.

At lunch that Sunday, my sister-in-law Edie leaned into my ear. "Pass the salt!" she whispered loudly. "It's right there, what's the matter with you?" I never liked Edie. She's so abrupt. But the salt *was* sitting right in front of me. Plain as day. I just didn't see it. When I drove home I noticed that the road signs still seemed hazy. I kept thinking, "I must need new glasses." So I went to my ophthalmologist the very next week.

"You have to see a retinal specialist," he said. He didn't sound urgent, just very matter of fact. The next Tuesday at nine A.M. I went to see the retinal specialist.

"Well," he said, all upbeat, "you've got macular degeneration. You have some irreversible vision loss, but most importantly, you need laser surgery right now to prevent additional loss. Can someone else drive you home?"

I just stared at him. *"What?"* was all I could say. I felt like I was hearing him through twelve feet of water. He kept talking, but I don't think I heard a word he said after "irreversible vision loss." My mind just froze on those words. I was so shocked.

After the laser surgery I think my vision was actually worse in my left eye. Several days later, I saw the specialist again. He seemed pleased.

"They're fine," he announced, "I think we've got it checked."

"Checked?" I said. "What about my vision? What happened to my vision?"

He didn't seem concerned. "That's to be expected," he said. "Hopefully you'll still keep some of your vision this way. Just stop driving. You won't go blind from this so you'll be okay." He patted me on the arm, and out he went. Just like that. Just like he was telling me Hudson's department store was having a summer sale on whites. With that much feeling.

But how am I going to be okay if I stop driving? I live in the metro Detroit area. You can't do anything without driving. All my friends live off different freeway exits. Do you realize that I'd have to walk two miles on roads without sidewalks where people are driving forty-five miles an hour *and* cross two six-lane intersections in order to get a carton of milk? How could he tell me I'm going to be fine and just walk out? How could he?

GRACE'S EXPERIENCE

Not everyone has Grace's experience. Many people feel very supported and encouraged by their doctors, especially those who receive visual rehabilitation program referrals and low vision resource information. On the other hand, a few people have experiences that are even worse than Grace's. One woman and her daughter recently told me that the specialist they had initially seen suggested she'd soon be blind from ARMD and then abruptly moved on to the next appointment. That sort of consultation is callous and incorrect. Macular degeneration does not cause blindness. It causes low vision. There is a difference. Fortunately, experiences like that aren't too common. But Grace's experience is common. Many times have I heard Grace's question, "How could he tell me I'm going to be fine and just walk out? How could he?" or "How could she?" Why? Are most doctors uncaring? No. Actually, most doctors care a great deal about their patients. They went into the field because they wanted to help people, and they work very hard to do their best. Even Grace's doctor was probably extremely competent, earnest, and well meaning. The problem is that many doctors have no idea how to communicate. They certainly weren't trained to talk to their patients, as strange as that might seem.

Why Doctors Aren't Always Good Communicators

In most medical programs, doctors are trained to isolate and treat physical problems the way an aeronautical engineer isolates and fixes problems on the space shuttle. They are trained under very stressful work conditions with long hours and little consideration for their own physical, emotional, or personal lives. They must learn to ignore these things for themselves, focus on problem solving, and move quickly. Their achievements and often their own sense of professional worthiness are measured by how well they fix the physical problem they were trained to fix, not by how well they relate to their patients or by how well they understand the implications of the problem for their patients' lives. When doctors are faced with a problem that they cannot really fix, like macular degeneration, they are faced with their own limitations. And they don't always know how to handle it sensitively.

Doctors who communicate well and offer their patients empathy, guidance, and options had to learn how to do that on their own, or were lucky enough to have supportive mentors. This is true even in specialties that often deal with death or conditions that bring major life changes. Eight years ago, my mother checked into a hospital near my parents' home with minor chest pain. The staff assured us that she was fine, but she stayed overnight for tests. Sometime in the early morning she suffered an unexpected heart attack. My father and I waited anxiously at the hospital for news. Eventually, a senior resident came out, stiffened, and blurted, "The code blue was unsuccessful." My father nodded gravely, stood up, and said, "Well, is she awake now? When can I see her?" The young doctor looked stunned. He had no idea what to say next. He had no idea how to tell my father that his beloved wife of fifty-three years had just died. He used the only language he was taught, which is what many doctors do.

Fortunately, some medical programs are beginning to focus on communication, but there is another impediment to supportive doctor-patient relationships. Practicing doctors are often squeezed by time constraints. Health costs dictate that they now need to see more patients than they did twenty years ago. Seeing more patients necessarily means spending less time with each patient, which means less time for addressing anything beyond the immediate diagnosis. Low vision rehabilitation for seniors is also a relatively new field. While most doctors would feel remiss if they failed to refer a stroke patient for physical rehabilitation, many doctors don't realize the importance of referring their low vision patients for visual rehabilitation.

The Importance of Early Visual Rehabilitation

Unfortunately, when doctors leave their patients without any empathetic recognition of the shock of macular degeneration, without any information on visual rehabilitation programs, and without resource or support group information, as Grace's doctor did, their patients often feel abandoned. They assume that there isn't any help available. If you have macular degeneration, having your experience recognized and hearing options for action, education, and support are critical for overcoming shock, and for handling the future. Low vision still isn't easy, but without any help it's much harder. If your doctor doesn't tell you about visual rehabilitation programs and resources in your area, ask. You can also contact the national organizations listed in the back of this book for programs. If there are no programs in your area, Part III of this book was designed for you. You can also use it to supplement your local program.

How Shock Interrupts Understanding

Often, when doctors do talk, we can't hear them. Just as Grace said that she didn't hear anything her doctor said after he told her she had

TIPS FOR TALKING WITH YOUR DOCTOR

1. Brainstorm your questions before your appointment, write them down, and take them with you.

2. Take a friend or family member along so there are two sets of ears listening in the room.

3. If you have difficulty understanding your doctor's explanations, ask if there is an assistant in the office who can explain in greater detail.

4. Ask your doctor for rehabilitation program information, resources, and low vision support groups in your area.

5. If you choose to order magnifiers from the consumer catalogs listed in the appendices, show these catalogs to your doctor, request advice, and use Chapter 12 for additional help.

6. Don't take it personally if your doctor isn't emotionally communicative or seems rushed. It is not a reflection of your condition or your potential.

"irreparable vision loss," it's often difficult for anyone to assimilate anything said after a shock. Our minds protect us emotionally by tuning out information that overwhelms us. Sometimes we don't even realize we've tuned out. We just don't remember that anything was said. I often find myself repeating information upon request, knowing that it's natural for people to have difficulty digesting it all at once. It's also easy to forget questions while you're at your doctor's office. To help your doctor help you, consider writing down a list of questions you may have and taking them to your appointment. Write large enough for you to see, in black felt tip or ink pen on white paper.

BEYOND SHOCK: ZELDA'S AND SAM'S EXPERIENCES

Just as people have different experiences of vision with macular degeneration, and different experiences of finding out about their decreased vision, they also have different experiences coping. We left Grace at a moment of crisis. After visiting her doctor, she felt so overwhelmed with the enormity of losing her driver's license, with fears of blindness, and with the apparent lack of help that she withdrew socially and struggled with depression for two years. Grace's depression lifted when she moved to a socially active senior community, came to visual rehabilitation, received some counseling, and joined a support group. "I used to daydream about running my doctor over with my Lincoln," Grace admitted frankly. "I never would have imagined that I'd say something like that, but for a long time macular degeneration took the graciousness out of me. Now I've started a new life." Like Grace, Zelda Grant also faced shock, but Zelda's fiery personality and her doctor's support made the experience different for her. Sam Weinberg, on the other hand, never really felt shocked. He was diagnosed with dry macular degeneration fifteen years ago, and his vision loss progressed very slowly, giving Sam plenty of time to adjust. Macular degeneration has, however, caused Sam to question his approach to life. He has worked to cultivate his sense of humor, which has helped him adjust to macular degeneration.

ZELDA GRANT'S STORY

The day my doctor told me that I had low vision from macular degeneration, I came home and smashed every dish in the house. All twelve place settings, two platters, and a cake plate. They were white china with little blue flowers that looked like little squiggly bugs to me. At the time, I was crying and screaming and smashing. There were chips everywhere, the kitchen floor was a mess. When I was done, all I had left were a half dozen navy-blue plastic bowls and a few coffee mugs, but I saved my life. If I hadn't smashed those dishes I'd be an angry woman with a pretty dining room setting that I couldn't really see anyway. I was angry for a long time as it was, and I sometimes still am, but smashing those dishes was a turning point, a declaration. I am going to live, and worrying about little blue flower-bugs on my plates is not a part of living anymore. Besides, if I hadn't smashed those plates it never would have occurred to me to get brightly colored plastic daily dishes that are easier to see and harder to break. The navy-blue bowls gave me that idea. On a white tablecloth, they are much more visible than white china ever could be.

So after I cleaned up my kitchen, I went through the information packet my doctor gave me, and began to make some phone calls. I called a rehabilitation program in my area and I said, "Hello. My name is Zelda Grant. I want an appointment, and I want to know how I'm going to keep reading." And then I called the neighborhood community center and I said, "Hello. My name is

Zelda Grant. I have low vision and I think I have a lot of energy. I need an exercise class." And then I called the support group listed in my information packet, and I said, "Hello. My name is Zelda Grant. What do you people talk about anyway?" I didn't bank on much to start with, but the more calls I made, and the more people I talked to, the easier it was to get help, and to do the things I wanted to do. You know, there are many people with inspiring approaches to life. I recently heard a quote from a paraplegic man named Mark Wellman who climbed a mountain at Yosemite National Park. Can you imagine climbing a mountain without using your legs? He says, "You have a dream and you know the only way that dream is going to happen is if you do it . . . even if it's six inches at a time." Now that's even a little much for me. I have a simpler motto. I just say, no matter who you are, if you stop trying you're dead. You just forgot to lie down.

SAM WEINBERG'S STORY

I first learned I had dry macular degeneration fifteen years ago. My doctor said, "Sam, you've got drusen here, but just a very slight amount of vision loss." I immediately thought, "My God, what's going to happen to my law practice?" I have a small-town private practice, mostly estate planning and compensation. I really worried that as soon as everyone knew, they'd decide they didn't want a visually impaired attorney. So I did everything I could to camouflage my low vision. I didn't even tell Rachel initially. I pretended I could see everything. I stayed up late at night using a magnifier and a bright desk lamp to read small-print documents and memorize them, so I could quote them verbatim and I wouldn't have to refer to papers during meetings. When new clients came, I called my secretary into the office and asked her to take detailed notes, type them, and print them in large font, so I wouldn't have to take notes myself. I stopped trying to read tiny price labels in the grocery store. I just took a lot of money with me and paid whatever the total came out to be. Rachel got suspicious pretty quickly. One day she eyed me and said, "You used to love coupons. What happened?"

After a few years, I just couldn't keep it a secret any longer, especially when my vision got worse. Rachel said, "Sam, they know you. They know you're a good lawyer. You're still a good lawyer." I didn't believe her at first, but she was right. My regular clients have been really loyal. They consult with me about ongoing issues, and bring me new cases. I also do a fair amount of consulting to younger attorneys, especially in the compensation field, since I know so much at this point. I work forty hours a week. And I spend a lot of time reading relevant journals and keeping up on the field. I have CCTVs for my office and my home, I have big-print software for my computer, and a large monitor. I use tape recorders for important meetings and depositions, I use floodlights in my office, and I write everything with thick black felt-tip pens. My secretary has gotten really adept at a low vision legal practice.

Sometimes I think Rachel would prefer it if I weren't working so hard. Actually, I've been thinking about cutting back because I'd like to spend more time with my violin. When I was young, I wanted to be a professional musician, but it didn't seem financially feasible. I figure now's my chance to play all the time!

Low vision has challenged me to be less earnest. I'm an overachiever, and that's gotten me far in life. But sometimes I forget to have a good time. So I've really tried to strengthen my sense of humor, and not take it all too seriously. Rachel keeps me on my toes. We went to a big party last week. Rachel wore a pair of distinctive black and white patent-leather shoes. She disappeared into the crowd, so I went looking for her shoes. When I thought I'd found them, I leaned over, puckered up, and whispered, "Are you my wife?" This woman jumped six inches, and huffed, "I certainly hope not!" "Too bad," I said, "You don't know what you're missing!" At the same party, I ate dry cat food. It was sitting in a bowl on the kitchen counter looking just like mixed nuts and pretzels. Rachel said, "Sam! What am I going to do with you?" And we laughed so hard we had tears in our eyes.

CHAPTER 6

With the Heart
One Sees Rightly:
Living Fully with ARMD

It is with the heart that one sees rightly; what is essential is invisible to the eye.

—Antoine de Saint-Exupéry
<u>The Little Prince</u>

I have met many people in the last few years, people whose courage matches their despair, whose hearts are still hopeful, people who are both defiant and defeated, angry and optimistic, fearful and faithful. As Bette Davis put it, "Growing old ain't for sissies." And neither is macular degeneration. But seniors are hardly sissies. If you are in your nineties, by the time you were half that old you had experienced two world wars and the greatest depression in the history of this country. If you are in your eighties, you barely remember the first war but you spent your teen years in the depression, and your young adulthood in the second war. If you are in your seventies, you missed the first war entirely, you just made the second one, and then you got to send your son to Vietnam. You grew up without social security, penicillin, civil rights, Title IX, Alcoholics Anonymous, Dr. Spock, or permanent press. And that's not easy. If you are in your sixties, you have just discovered, on the eve of your retirement, that you are losing your vision, with twenty or thirty years of living ahead of you. And that's not easy either.

You have probably already experienced profound losses in your life, but losing vision is a new kind of loss. Unlike deaths, accidents, or serious illnesses, ARMD comes quietly, often without public recognition, certainly without flowers or phone calls. It doesn't seem very dramatic, until it happens to you. As Buddy Burmester said, "You wouldn't believe how often you use your eyes every day for everything. But it's not just that I can't see what I want to see. It affects my sense of control over my life, and my confidence with other people. It affects everything. I guess I assumed my eyes would always be there for me."

Since vision loss is a new kind of loss, it raises new issues and requires new coping skills which may be unfamiliar to you. They include:

- expressing your feelings

- addressing depression

- joining the macular degeneration community

- seeing your potential positively, and gaining skills and confidence through visual rehabilitation

- exercising for better health and living

- taking risks

EXPRESSING YOUR FEELINGS

For many people, losing vision is like losing a loved one. You may have very strong feelings about your vision loss: feelings of anger, frustration, fear, regret, embarrassment, or grief. Vision loss deserves grieving and acknowledgment. You don't have to smash plates like Zelda Grant, but give yourself permission to feel strongly, and permission to express your feelings. Expressing your feelings means identifying how you feel and sharing your feelings in all of their depth and richness to a friend, family member, religious advisor, or counselor. Some people even share their feelings with their pets. Others turn to a patron saint. Turn to someone with whom you feel comfortable, someone who will listen supportively and acknowledge your feelings.

Just as there are many different people to whom you may turn, there are also many different ways of expressing your feelings. Expressing your feelings may mean crying, screaming, whispering, writing, dancing, walking, just plain old talking, or punching a bed pillow. Expressing your feelings may also be a process that unfolds over time, and through many conversations. Zelda didn't accept having low vision in one afternoon. I doubt anyone does. Whatever you do, though, don't bottle yourself up and tell yourself that you don't really have a reason to have feelings at all.

"Express your feelings" may be advice that makes sense to you, but it may not. If you are over sixty-five, you were probably raised to be polite and to keep private matters private. Women in senior generations were taught to make others comfortable whenever possible. Men were taught that feelings are a sign of weakness. And everyone was taught to get tough and pull themselves up by the bootstraps. Feelings weren't even really a topic of public conversation until the baby boomers became the Me generation. Before 1965, feelings were things you had about your first crush. Having too many of them wasn't generally considered a good idea. They might get in the way of meeting your responsibilities at work or at home. But the fact that you don't show your feelings doesn't mean you don't have them. And if you don't acknowledge them, they may weigh heavily on you or they may erupt in other areas of your life, or you may spend so much energy keeping them in check that you aren't really free to feel fully alive or face the future.

Pulling Yourself Up by the Bootstraps

So does expressing your feelings mean you shouldn't pull yourself up by the bootstraps? Is bootstrapping a thing of the past? Absolutely not. It's still a good thing. But today's bootstrapping is different from yesterday's. Pulling yourself up by the bootstraps used to mean doing it all alone. It used to mean having as few needs and as few feelings as possible. It used to mean being carefully dignified and keeping a stiff upper lip. It used to mean saving your money in order to buy white gloves for Sundays or shopping downtown. But the world has changed in the last thirty years. Now we wear sweatpants to the airport and the doctor's office, neighbors and friends talk openly about coping with breast cancer and alcoholism, and strangers reveal their private lives on television. As a society, we've taken off the white gloves. But as individuals, we often keep them close at hand. We still cling to the idea that coping well means being quiet, and dignity means doing things properly the first time. But that's not true, and it's an idea that isn't doing us any favors.

Redefining Bootstrapping

Zelda Grant was bootstrapping when she had a screaming fit in her kitchen and smashed all her plates. She was bootstrapping when she called for a visual rehabilitation appointment, and when she called her neighborhood club to enroll in an exercise class. And she was bootstrapping when she called her local low vision support group and said, "Hello. My name is Zelda Grant. What do you people talk about anyway?" She may not be winning any points for tact or diplomacy, but as a bootstrapper she's a champion. Bootstrapping today means having feelings, figuring out what they are, and expressing them. Bootstrapping today means having needs, figuring out what they are, and getting them met. Bootstrapping today means asking for the support you need and learning the skills that will enable you to do as much as you can.

Most importantly, though, bootstrapping today means putting the white gloves away. It means taking the risk that you won't do it properly the first time, that you won't avoid every spill, that you won't always look absolutely perfect. And it means realizing that that's okay. Bootstrapping means putting on your finest clothes for a dinner party and chuckling when you realize you've served paper towels in the tossed salad. Because the truth is that nobody really minds. People like you for you, not for what you can see. Bootstrapping means enjoying their company and realizing that the greatest dignity of all comes from just living.

DEPRESSION AND MACULAR DEGENERATION

Many people who lose vision go through a short period of mild depression as they grieve their loss and adjust their lives. But many others experience prolonged periods of depression that are unhealthy for the body and spirit. We know a great deal more about depression than we did twenty or thirty years ago. We know that it's not a sign of weakness, laziness, or moral failure. We know that depression happens to people who have no other psychological difficulties. We know that depression can happen to you later in life even if you've never been depressed before. And we know that depression is very common among people with low vision. There is nothing shameful about it, but there is something very tragic about living with depression without getting help.

Common Symptoms of Depression

Consider the list below and ask yourself whether or not any of these symptoms are familiar.

- Frequently feeling apathetic or unmotivated

- Frequently feeling agitated, empty, or numb

- Feeling negatively about yourself or frequently pessimistic

- Withdrawing socially

- Insomnia or hypersomnia (sleeping too little or too much)

- Losing or gaining more than 5 percent of your body weight in a month

- Noticeable decrease in energy

- Unexplained episodes of crying

What Causes Depression with Macular Degeneration?

Depression with macular degeneration may arise from deep feelings of rage, grief, or frustration, from isolation or loneliness, from prolonged inactivity or boredom, from self-judgment, from fearing the future, or from feeling out of control or without options. Some people may be genetically predisposed to depression. Your diet and exercise patterns may also make a difference. If you live in a car-centered area without good public transportation, like most of the Midwest and many suburbs, and you lose your driver's license, you may also be more likely to experience depression. Losing your license may initially contribute to isolation and loneliness, especially if you've always relied on cars. It may also affect your sense of independence and personal style. That doesn't mean that everyone who lives in the Midwest becomes depressed when they get low vision, or that New Yorkers never get depressed with low vision, but losing your driver's license can be a major blow.

Why You Can't Always Strong-Arm Your Way Out

Many seniors make the mistake of thinking they should strong-arm their way out of depression. Worse, they think that if they can't strong-arm their way out, there's something wrong with them. Worst of all, they think they just have to live with it. People often come to my office to talk about their low vision. They say, "Well, I guess I just have to make the best of it," then set their jaws, and look away. Sometimes, the gentlest people cry, and sometimes the proudest people cry, as Grace Olsen did. They don't mean they have to make the best of low vision. They mean they have to make the best of being *depressed* with low vision. But depression is not something you want to put up with and embrace as a partner in life. It's bad for your physical health, your emotional health, and your spirit. Depression can also negatively affect your relationships with other people and strain your marriage. Don't decide that you just have to make the best of depression. And don't camouflage it.

There are two reasons why you may not be able to strong-arm your way out of depression, and neither of them has anything to do with being weak. First, depression is a real physiological condition, not just a mindset or a bad attitude. Research suggests that stressful situations and significant losses in our lives affect the production and regulation of chemicals in our brains that influence our emotional state and our immune system. Once you are depressed, you may remain depressed if you do not receive professional help and take direct action, because the balance of chemicals in your brain may actually promote your depression, or at least sustain it. Second, if your depression was triggered by loneliness, isolation, or inactivity, it is unlikely to lift from thinking alone. You need to address the root of the problem.

Treating Depression

The more you do, the better. The first thing you should do, however, is talk to your doctor. Then act on the following suggestions with his or her advice.

- Ask your doctor about antidepressant medications and alternative treatments like St. John's Wort. St. John's Wort is a mild herbal remedy used for depression that is very popular in Europe and may have fewer side effects than regular medications. It may also be less expensive. However, it may affect your blood pressure.

- If you are sensitive to sugar or alcoholism runs in your family, ask your doctor about switching to a balanced carbohydrate-protein diet that is designed to keep your glucose levels stable. Diet may contribute to depression in some people.

- Begin a regular routine of physical exercise (follow the suggestions under "Living Through Exercising" below). Exercise has been shown to be an effective remedy for depression in many people. It actually acts on the chemicals in our brains to help stabilize our moods. Exercise also has many other health benefits.

- Attend a visual rehabilitation program in your area. If your doctor does not know of one, call the organizations listed in Appendix I for information. If there is no program in your area, follow Part III of this book.

- If you live with family or alone, make an effort to cultivate your own commitments, activities, interests, and friends. Making new friends as a senior may seem difficult, especially if you've had the same friends for years and you're out of practice, and low vision doesn't make it easier. But when friends move or pass away, or when your husband or wife dies, it's really important to reconnect with others. And you can do it. Loneliness and isolation are not good for you. You must do whatever you can to avoid them. You may want to consider moving into a socially active senior residence if at all possible, someplace where you can make friends and be involved.

- Find and use alternative modes of transportation. Contact your local transportation authority for bus, rail, or subway information. Call taxi cab companies and ask about their service and rates (see Chapter 14). If you are used to driving your own car, you may balk at paying bus or cab fares. However, the cost of buses and cabs may be equal to—or less than—the cost of maintaining your car, especially when you count insurance. And remember, outside of the convenience of owning a car, there is nothing inherently special about driving yourself around; the richest people in the world have chauffeurs.

- Seek professional counseling, especially counseling that complements visual rehabilitation by helping you express your feelings, focus on your skills, and combat self-judging or limiting thoughts.

YOU ARE IN GOOD COMPANY: THE ARMD COMMUNITY

The macular degeneration community in America has millions of members. If you have macular degeneration, you are in good company. You may be sixty or you may be one hundred. You may be a homemaker, a small businessowner, journalist, national master's swimmer, retired trucker, engineer, parent, grandparent or great-grandparent, a famous painter like Georgia O'Keeffe, or a former first lady like Lady Bird Johnson. You may have just discovered you have macular degeneration, or you may have been living with it for decades. Whoever you are, and whatever your vision, there are many, many people in America who share this condition with you. They're right in your neighborhood. And they're all across the country, too.

In the last few years, people with low vision from macular degeneration have begun to write about their experiences, reaching out to others with low vision and telling the world the way it is. Journalist Henry Grunwald wrote his memoir "Losing Sight" for *The New Yorker*. He continues to write. Professor Carolyn See wrote a personal essay for *Modern Maturity*, the magazine of the American Association of Retired People (AARP). Bert Silverman of Portland, Maine published *Bert's Eye View: Coping with Macular Degeneration* in 1997, and two large-print classics, Nicolette Pernot Ringgold's *Out of the Corner of My Eye: Living With Vision Loss in Later Life* and Frances Neer's *Dancing in the Dark* are also in print. You'll find these articles and books listed at the end of the Selected Bibliography.

There are also two associations for ARMD,

both founded by people with low vision from macular degeneration. The Association for Macular Diseases (AMD) is an international support group founded twenty years ago for people with macular disease and their families. AMD maintains a telephone hot line for members, publishes a newsletter with information on current research, conducts nationwide seminars on ARMD, and has offices in New York and Philadelphia. Nikolai Stevenson, who has macular degeneration, has been the president of AMD for the past fifteen years. You can join AMD by calling 212-605-3719 or writing to the address listed in the Appendix. Macular Degeneration International was founded by Tom Perski in Tucson, Arizona, seven years ago. Like AMD, MDI now has members worldwide. MDI publishes a newsletter which includes low vision resource information. You can join MDI by calling 520-797-2525 or writing to the address in the Appendix.

Join a Support Group

Joining a support group is a very powerful way to be a part of your community. It can also be a great experience. Some people assume that support groups are only for people with talkative personalities, or those who can't cope on their own. But that's not true. Support groups are for everyone. Lots of people who don't have low vision have a support group, they just don't call it that. For example, Rotary Clubs, Lions Clubs, chambers of commerce, and small business associations are all support groups. They are places to share a common experience, get advice and tips, network and meet others, and avoid having to reinvent the wheel on your own. Try it, you'll like it. Call your local rehabilitation program for support group information, ask your doctor for a referral, or call the national organizations listed in the back of this book. They may be able to connect you with a group in your area.

Start Your Own Support Group

If there is no support group in your area, it doesn't mean there aren't any seniors with low vision in your area, it just means that no one is getting the benefit of a support group. Everyone is reinventing the wheel all by themselves, and feeling very alone doing it. Why not start a group? Use the suggestions below as handy guidelines:

- To find potential members, ask your local clergy to announce a new support group or put an announcement in a newsletter or bulletin. Make a large-print flyer to post or distribute at local churches, synagogues and mosques. Include your phone number so potential members can call and ask questions.

- Call your local paper and ask them to

interview you about living with macular
degeneration and profile your efforts to start
a support group.

- Call your local senior center and ask them to
announce your new group in their
membership information. Send them big-
print flyers to post and distribute.

- A support group can be as small as two
people, and as large as you would like it to
be. If your group starts out with two, don't be
disappointed, more will join if you let them
know you're meeting.

- You can hold your support group in your
home, in other members' homes, or ask for
available free space at a house of worship or
community center. You may want to decide
on a meeting place after you know who the
members may be and where they live so you
can choose the most convenient location for
everyone.

- Collect public transportation information
for members, arrange car pools or shared
taxis.

- Most groups meet once or twice a month.
In general, it's best to set a regular
meeting time, like the first Monday of
the month at one P.M., so that members can

plan ahead. You may want to make this decision as a group after you meet for the first time.

- You can choose a topic for each meeting ahead of time, or simply go around the circle and see if anyone has an experience, question, or answer to share. You can also use this book as a framework for your discussions by reading a personal story from Part II: Experiencing ARMD or a tip from Part III. You may also want to invite guest speakers.

- When you first meet, set some ground rules as a group. Here are a few suggestions from the National Association for the Visually Handicapped (NAVH), which conducts workshops and provides resources for groups nationwide:

  —Always introduce yourself when you enter the room, and introduce new people to everyone present.
  —Avoid whispering. Speak clearly enough so everyone can hear.
  —Speak up if you don't hear someone clearly.
  —If your group talks about private matters, like relationships with spouses, keep a confidentiality rule. Everything said in the group stays in the group.

THE STORIES WE HEAR AND THE STORIES WE TELL

New books constantly arrive on bookstore shelves or on cassette tapes that talk to, for, or about seniors. There are new memoirs, like Carolyn Heilbrun's *The Last Gift of Time: Life Beyond Sixty*; there are new philosophies, like Rabbi Salman Schachter-Shalomi's *From Age-ing to Sage-ing: A Profound New Vision of Growing Older*; and there are new reports on health, like *Successful Aging: The MacArthur Foundation Study*. Although each book takes a different approach, they all tell the same truth: that being a senior is a stage of life as important as every other stage. Seniors are a growing part of American society. Even though we may not have the bodies we used to have, we can do much more than we often assume we can, mentally *and* physically. And that's true of seniors with low vision, too.

That's much different from the story people were telling each other twenty years ago. Twenty years ago, "disengagement theory" was popular. Disengagement theory held that as you became a senior, regardless of your own desires, you should reduce your activities, interests, and your list of friends. The idea was that limiting yourself made accepting death easier. Not surprisingly, doctors have discovered that disengaging doesn't do much except make you miserable. In fact, they not only discovered that disengaging is bad for you, but that engaging is good for you. Pursuing the activities you enjoy, keeping and making new friends, and following a regular physical exercise routine can actually improve your memory and your mood, strengthen your balance and your stamina, boost your immune system, and increase your overall quality of life. And it doesn't matter if you're exercising in a wheelchair or if you start when you're ninety. You can still reap the benefits of engaging.

The Stories We Tell About Ourselves

Just as doctors and public policy makers tell stories about what it means to be older, we also tell stories about what it means to be ourselves. Sometimes we don't even realize we are telling stories. But realize it or not, the stories we tell about ourselves are enormously influential, especially when we believe them. One of the most common stories people tell me about themselves is that they are less appealing and have less to offer others because they have low vision. "I don't go down to the dining room for lunch anymore because I'm afraid I'll spill coffee on myself," Rosa Garcia admitted quietly. "And besides, I can't see people too well so I'm not sure I'll have much to say." After I talked with Rosa for a while, I discovered that she has opinions about the president and bilingual education, and she loves the Chicago White Sox. She has a wonderfully warm smile, and sixty years' experience as a mother, grand-mother, and parish secretary. Why wouldn't anyone want to talk with her?

The Power of Positive Stories

Inspirational speakers like Norman Vincent Peale and Dale Carnegie, and religious leaders like Billy Graham have been telling us for decades that positive thinking is powerful. That's why every major religious tradition teaches love and forgiveness, because these are the two most powerful stories of living: that we love and are loved, and that we forgive the foibles of ourselves and others. Listen to the positive stories you hear about seniors in the world and tell positive stories about yourself and about what you can do. We're all human; we all have doubts, insecurities, and embarrassments. We always will. But don't make them the only truth in your life.

WHEN STORIES COME TO LIFE

The inspiring guide *Secrets of Becoming a Late Bloomer* encourages all seniors to be as active as they can, doing the things they want to do. The book tells the story of Jack who has macular degeneration and becomes a reading tutor for children. Jack's the third person I've found with low vision from ARMD who tutors reading. It's a brilliant idea, actually. In Jack's case, he decided that he'd always liked children, so he contacted a volunteer placement service. They sent him to meet with the local elementary school principal. The principal told Jack that what the school really needed was reading tutors, but she assumed that Jack's low vision meant he couldn't help. "I suppose the idea's completely out of the question," she concluded. But Jack explained that the children could read to him aloud and he would correct their pronunciation. If a child couldn't read a word, Jack would ask him or her to spell it aloud, and would help the child figure out the word. This tutoring strategy works well for Jack and his students, and it works well for other people with low vision who also tutor reading. When I read Jack's story, I realized I was not only reading the story of someone's experience, but I was also reading about how Jack managed to tell a different story about his potential than the one the principal assumed was true. And I realized that Jack's story illustrates visual rehabilitation at its best.

Visual Rehabilitation

As you'll discover when you turn to Part III of this book, visual rehabilitation is about learning new skills, like reading with low vision, and using new products, like magnifiers, halogen light bulbs, and CCTVs. Those are the nuts and bolts. At its heart, though, visual rehabilitation is really about saying, "Hey world, this is what I need and this is what I'd like to do," and then not taking *no* for an answer, at least not easily. It's about telling your own story of what you can do, rather than listening to someone else's.

As you already know, telling your own story isn't always easy. Macular degeneration can turn the world upside down, making the familiar seem unfamiliar, and the safe feel precarious. It can make you much more aware of what you can't do than what you can do. Macular degeneration can make living in your community seem like traveling in a foreign country without the glamour of flying somewhere. If you're in Greece, ordering dinner at a restaurant when you can't read the local language is exotic and exciting, but it loses its appeal if it happens in your hometown. Visual rehabilitation is about turning the world right side up again, making it safe, and making it work for you. Visual rehabilitation is about putting more things in the "can do" column than the "can't do" and developing the tools to tell your own story. After all, Jack makes volunteer tutoring look simple, but he had to get to the elementary school somehow, and he had to have a bit of confidence to stand up and explain how he was going to tutor reading without having his central vision. Where did those skills come from? They came from visual rehabilitation.

Telling Your Own Story

The story you tell about yourself or what you'd like to do doesn't have to be the same as Jack's. Not everyone wants to be a reading tutor or volunteer in any capacity (although the rewards can be invaluable). When I asked Rosa Garcia what she would like to do, she said she'd like to make dinner for her family. My father likes to bowl. Grace Olsen likes to play bridge with a few friends using big-print cards. Sam and Rachel Weinberg like to go to the opera; they also enjoy traveling to elder hostel courses. Zelda likes to raise Cain in her yoga class, her support group, and her book club (she listens to books on tape, while the other members read regular paperbacks). Your own story can be whatever you want it to be, but make it about living fully in whatever ways you would most enjoy.

LIVING THROUGH EXERCISING

If you are older and have low vision, you may assume that you can't exercise or that it wouldn't be safe. Not true! Actually, exercise is really important for people with macular degeneration, because low vision often reduces your activity and mobility. If you don't make an effort, you may become more sedentary, and that's not good for your overall health. Exercise improves your stamina and balance; it helps stabilize sleep patterns and insulin levels; it improves your outlook and mood; and it improves the length and quality of your life. Not only that, but you don't have to be an athlete to reap the benefits of exercise. You just have to start exercising. The hardest part of exercising, however, is starting. The next hardest part is sticking with it for at least one month. After a month, your body will become more accustomed to exercising and you will feel better on a daily basis, even before you start seeing changes in your body. Stay with a program for at least six months to a year. If you stop, you can begin again and still benefit. Your body is remarkably elastic; you just have to give it a chance. You will see changes.

Always check with your doctor before you begin an exercise program. Begin modestly, and increase your program gradually. If you are not accustomed to exercising, begin with five minutes of walking or riding an exercycle four to five times a week. When this becomes easy, increase your time gradually, until you reach twenty to thirty minutes a day four to five times a week. Talk to your doctor about adding gentle stretches to your program to loosen the muscles that you use and prevent injury. If you cannot walk, consider lifting leg or arm weights. You can buy lightweight ones with Velcro straps for your ankles and wrists, or you can hold light arm weights.

If you are worried about falling, talk with your doctor. Ask about walking with a cane or with a friend or workout partner, riding a stationary bike, lifting weights while sitting, or exercising in a pool with assistance.

SUGGESTIONS FOR EXERCISING

- Take gentle yoga, stretching, or tai chi classes. Ask the instructor to give clear verbal directions (they usually do anyway) and don't worry about how well you're doing. Just do it.

- Join a senior-friendly workout club or YMCA. Use their stationary bikes, rowing machines, and weight machines. Ask about weight training classes and personal programs. You can also buy a stationary bike or rowing machine for your home. Use hand-held weights or Velcro-strap weights at home to strengthen your arms and legs.

- Swim, kick across the pool with a kickboard, or use an aqua-jogger belt to run upright in the pool. You can buy one at a local sports store. If you can't swim or would like to exercise with other people, take a water aerobics class.

- Walk.

TAKING RISKS

People tend to recognize physical risks as risks, but they don't always talk about social risks as risks. Those slide under the table. But social risks are a big concern for many people with macular degeneration. No one avoids them. My father has asked a mannequin for directions to the men's department, taken the wrong bus, hugged a stranger, passed by old friends on the street, and missed bowling pins. But none of these mistakes have cost him friends or dignity. The answer to almost any social situation is to be straightforward about your vision, and remember that fears are *fears*, not reflections of what will really happen or what others will really think.

Keep Your Sense of Humor

If you can see the risks of low vision with a light-hearted eye, at least sometimes, they become much less pressing. Francie Klein, who is a marvelous cook, recently made cherry pie for a party with kidney beans instead of cherries. "I had a good laugh about it," she said. "I'm lucky because my father taught me how to live with macular degeneration. He had it, too. He once took a bite out of a cork coaster, mistaking it for an almond cookie. "Dad!" I said, "that's a coaster!" "Well, thank goodness," he said. "I thought your cooking was going to pot."

Let Others Know You Have Low Vision

If you have macular degeneration, you won't look any different to anyone else. People may assume you can see them, and you may pass old friends on the street. Tell everyone you know that you have low vision and you may not recognize them. They have to say hello directly and introduce themselves. After a while, your friends and acquaintances will adjust. Newcomers may be temporarily confused, so you may always run into this problem. But anyone who gets upset because you didn't say hello first, or respond when they waved, needs to have their head examined. You can tell them I said so. Besides, they'll feel foolish if they get macular degeneration and need your advice. You may think I'm kidding, but I'm not. Whatever you do, though, don't squash your own personality with worry. Go get 'em.

Don't Hesitate to Ask for Assistance

Do everything you can for yourself, and don't hesitate to ask for assistance. That sounds like contradictory advice, but it's really not. Sometimes you need a bit of assistance to do something for yourself. Better to ask a store clerk to read a price tag than to avoid shopping altogether. Better to ask a pedestrian which bus is pulling up than to avoid public transportation. Better to ask a family member or friend if your lipstick is on right than to avoid going outside. This last example touches a sensitive spot for many people. If you've taken pride in your appearance all your life, as most of us have, you may feel chagrined to find out that you're wearing brown socks with a blue suit, or wearing a sweater that needs a trip to the cleaners. But let's be honest. It's not a character weakness to mismatch colors or have a piece of string or a spot on your clothes. Other people are unlikely to even notice; and if they do, they are unlikely to think anything of it at all. We always care more about our own appearance than anyone else does.

If you are very concerned, ask others to tell you if they notice anything amiss in your appearance. Remember, it's no different from fully sighted people having a smudge of chocolate on their face or a small mark on the back of their skirt. They rely on someone else to tell them, so ask them to tell you. Make a deal with your family, friends, and neighbors that you want them to tell you if they notice anything amiss in your appearance because it helps you to know. I made this deal with my father and we're both so used to it now, that we don't think twice. He feels more comfortable knowing I'll tell him, and I feel more comfortable knowing I can tell him.

Be Honest with Friends and Family

Dostoevsky once wrote that "much unhappiness has come into the world because of bewilderment and things left unsaid." I often talk with people who are reluctant to tell their friends and family much about their low vision for fear of distressing or burdening them. Sometimes they aren't being honest about small things. But sometimes those small things pile up and become big things. When Grace first lost her driver's license from low vision, she decided not to attend bridge club anymore because she couldn't drive herself. Since she would never know whether or not she would be a burden, Grace declined her friend Lily's offer of a ride. Besides, Grace reasoned, she couldn't see regular playing cards very well anyway and she didn't want to ask the group to play with big-print cards. For several weeks, Lily called her, but Grace held firm. Grace's stoic determination to remain independent was admirable, but misguided. She managed to make herself very lonely, and Lily, too.

I happen to know Lily, and know that she really enjoyed Grace's company and enjoyed having dinner with Grace after bridge club. "Grace won't come to bridge club anymore," Lily told me when I saw her outside the grocery store. "I guess her vision is going and she doesn't feel like playing cards. I tried to call her, but she won't come." There was something resigned and sad in Lily's voice. As she turned and walked away, I watched her tiny, sloping shoulders disappear down the street. Lily cares a lot more about Grace's company, I thought, than she does about whether or not Grace can drive herself to bridge club, and Grace isn't listening. Fortunately, Grace finally realized that she has more to offer her friends than perfect vision. Today Grace takes a cab to bridge club, the group plays with big-print cards, and Lily drives her home after they've had dinner together. And they are both happier. There is nothing independent about forcing yourself to stay home in order to avoid being dependent. Don't shut out your friends. Instead, tell them what you need, and look for alternative ways to do what you want to do.

Adapting to New Roles

Taking risks may also mean adapting to new roles for you and your family. "For fifty years I never drove," Inez Toscano exclaimed to me when her husband, Joe, came to the Low Vision Living Program at our center. "Imagine, at seventy-five I got my first driver's license! But since Joe can't drive, I needed one. It seems like a small thing, but it feels very strange." Sam and Rachel Weinberg found themselves adjusting to new roles, too. "We've always been very independent of one another," Sam said earnestly, "but now we often work as a team." Rachel winked and squeezed

Sam's hand affectionately. "Yes, it's teamwork. But it's also 'Rachel. Rachel! Could you double-check these figures please?! Rachel! Could you come and look at this please?' Rachel! Rachel! I might change my name to Veronica." Being honest about your feelings and needs will help make these adjustments easier for everyone.

LIVING WITH FAITH

When I first met Evangeline, who has low vision from macular degeneration, she told me a ribald joke. At ninety, she didn't miss a beat. After an hour, she announced that she couldn't stay any longer because she'd miss her luncheon date with her gentleman friend. "Have you any advice for the younger generation?" I asked, figuring that I could take the advice myself and be as vibrant in thirty years as she is today. She smiled and paused, clearly choosing her words.

"Yes," she finally said, "I will tell you what I tell my great-grandchildren. Pray to the holy family."

"That's it?" I said.

"Yes, that's it," she said. And out she went.

The holy family? Not being Catholic, I didn't see an immediate use for the advice. But as I met more and more people with low vision, I remembered Evangeline's words. I began to understand that faith plays an important part in how we experience life, and how we experience low vision. By faith I mean the belief that you are valuable as an individual, *no matter what,* and that your life has meaning. Faith protects us from unnecessary anxiety. Faith forgives us and makes sense of fate. Faith is also a muscle that we can exercise: it can grow strong through time and through engagement with the activities and people you enjoy.

Whatever faith you profess, I tell my patients, I have faith in you. You are our role models. We look to you, as I looked to Evangeline, to see how to handle being older and losing vision. You are the first generation to do so. And we're right behind you.

CHAPTER 7

Fifteen Tips
for Family and Friends

A faithful friend is the medicine of life.
—Ecclesiasticus 6:16

Many family members and friends of people with ARMD have asked me what they can do to help. Here are fifteen tips:

1. Be Direct About Vision

Ask your friend or family member what they can and can't see so that you know. Don't worry about using phrases that emphasize vision, like "Did you see Zelda yesterday?"

2. Identify Yourself and Say Hello

Take the initiative to say hello and identify yourself when you see your family member or friend. And don't always assume that other seniors can see you. At the very least, one out of every twelve seniors over seventy-five has low vision.

3. Give Clear Directions

Give clear verbal directions and avoid vague replies like "It's over there." Don't assume that your friend or family member can read your facial expressions or gestures. Say in words everything you want to convey.

4. Use Black Felt-Tip or Ink Pens and Print in Clear Lettering

Always write notes or letters to your family or friend in black felt tip or ink pen or black computer print. Print clearly in letters large enough for your friend or family member to see. Don't use colored paper or pens, ballpoint pens, or pencils since they are very difficult to see. For birthdays and holidays, consider calling instead of sending a card.

5. Give Low-Vision Gifts

Consider giving low-vision gifts like talking calculators, watches, clocks, thermometers, weight scales, or computer software. You could also give large-button or automatic dialing phones, large-print cards, clocks, calendars, or address books. There are all kinds of other gifts to choose from in the low-vision catalogs listed at the end of this book. Alternatively, consider giving a book on tape, tickets to a concert, or help purchase a CCTV.

6. Keep the Environment Predictable

A predictable environment makes a big difference for anyone with low vision. Many people can compensate for less vision by relying on their knowledge of the environment. Help your friend or family member keep their home (and yours if you live together) as predictable as possible. Keep frequently used items like house keys, salt shakers, and trash bags in designated places. Put things away after you use them, and close cupboard and stairwell doors. If you are a guest, return any item you move to the place you found it, even a coffee table book that looks merely decorative. If the color of the book contrasts with the coffee table, your friend or family member may be using it to see the coffee table more clearly.

7. Offer Your Arm, Don't Take Theirs

When you walk with your friend or family member, offer your arm. Don't take their arm because you may throw them off balance. This guideline for walking applies to all of low-vision life: offer help where it's necessary, but don't just do it yourself.

8. Don't Just Do for Your Parent

Enable your parent to do as much for him or herself as possible. Don't assume that because of low vision your parent isn't capable, and don't foster that assumption in your parent. If your parent wants to take out the trash, walk to the cleaner's, mow the lawn, cook a family dinner, volunteer at a local center, or run a manufacturing company, so much the better! As busy adult children, we often feel like less responsibility would be a relief for us, so that must be true for our parents. But having nothing to work toward can be deathly boring. Too much responsibility is stressful, but too little is unhealthy. Don't take away anyone's reason for having to be up and about in the morning. And don't take away anyone's ability to help you. Take the time you would have spent doing your parent's chores and share some activity you both enjoy.

9. Share Activities You Both Enjoy

Find new or old activities that please both of you. Call your friend or family member and make a date. Here are a few suggestions:

- Dine out.

- Attend a wine tasting or food fair.

- Go to the symphony or an opera concert.

- Go to a botanical garden.

- Golf, bowl, swim, lift weights, walk in a park.

- Listen to a book on tape or National Public Radio news together.

- Do a crossword puzzle together.

- Play cards, chess, checkers, or large-print scrabble.

- Demonstrate at a political rally.

- Get facials and manicures.

- Go to a lecture series, a book reading, or poetry reading.

- Go to a baseball or football game (you can also listen to commentary on the radio either at home or in the stadium).

- Take yoga, stretching classes, tai chi, water aerobics, or meditation classes.

- Start or join a salon, discussion group, or support group.

- Attend religious services.

- Volunteer at a local charity.

- Sail or skydive, with a qualified instructor, of course.

10. Encourage Interests

When you lose vision, you don't lose your physical or mental energy. Encourage your friend or family member to maintain old interests and cultivate new ones. Encourage hobbies, volunteer work, membership in senior clubs or support groups, and listening to National Public Radio news or to *Newsweek* on cassette tape. We so often think of paid jobs or parenting as significant, and hobbies or interests as optional, but they're not. Everybody needs to be a part of their community, aware of it, and alive in it. When you're younger, jobs and parenting may take up most of your time, but when you're a senior you have time for other interests. And whatever you spend your time doing is just as important for the quality of your life today as your job was for the quality of your life in earlier years. For adult children especially, retirement may look like heaven, and having no role may seem like sweet relief. But just being retired without any interests, or just living comfortably in a tidy apartment without much stimulation, or just coping with low vision as a full-time preoccupation is a short-term recipe for boredom, and a long-term recipe for personal distress and crisis. Being alive is the sum total of our actions, mental and physical, in this world. Be active, encourage action.

11. Realize the Importance of Friends

If you are a friend, realize how important you are. If you are an adult child, realize that everyone needs friends. We are so used to thinking of family as our fortress and friends as nice but not as necessary, that we may discount their importance. While family is often our fortress, friends may be equally so, and sometimes even more important for seniors' happiness and longevity. I often meet seniors who have moved out of their communities and into apartments in their adult children's neighborhoods. The move initially solves a number of problems: the adult child feels more confident caring for their parent, the parent feels safer, and keeping accurate banking records or troubleshooting with doctors may be easier. But over time, as the adult child returns to his or her responsibilities, working full time or shuttling children to school, the senior parent spends the vast majority of the day alone.

Without any friends, seniors are prone to loneliness *regardless of how much their adult children try to meet their needs*. And loneliness is not a good thing. It does not make you very excited about living, and may even lead to clinical depression. Keeping old friends and making new ones should be at the very top of the priority list when considering living arrangements. I strongly recommend that seniors stay connected to their local communities, move to senior residences that feature plenty of social events and encourage meeting people, or actively work to make new friends, join new groups, and engage in new activities with others wherever they move. Adult children would do their parents a greater service helping them make or keep friends than almost anything else.

12. Watch for Depression

Depression is very common among people with macular degeneration. Many people experience a short period of depression as they adjust to vision loss, but many others experience prolonged periods of depression. Be aware of changes in your friend or family member's emotional state, sleeping patterns, weight, or behavior. Excessive worry, bouts of crying, listlessness or disinterest, low motivation, pessimism or snippiness, social withdrawal, a refusal to communicate or an excessively stiff upper lip, moping, or helplessness may all signal depression. Depression is not healthy for anyone. See Chapter 6, and talk directly to your friend or family member about your concerns. If your spouse or parent appears depressed, make an appointment with his or her doctor, pursue visual rehabilitation, and get them out into the world or involved in new activities (even if you have to give a gentle push).

13. Participate in Visual Rehabilitation

Participating in visual rehabilitation in the broadest sense means fostering a sense of independence, self-determination, and joy. That does not mean that anyone who is successfully pursuing visual rehabilitation needs to prove that they can do it all by themselves, live on their own, or get a volunteer job. But it does mean living as fully as possible. There are many practical things you can do to help someone follow a program of visual rehabilitation. Here are just a few suggestions:

- Read a Visual Rehabilitation chapter together from Part III of this book and talk about implementing the suggestions.

- Do the reading workshop together.

- Help rearrange furniture, tape down area rugs, install new lighting fixtures, choose contrasting tablecloths or dishes.

- Help rearrange clothing on shelves for better visibility.

- Help label files, boxes, bottles, stove dials, washing machine dials, and canned goods.

- If you live together, tell your friend or family member what they can do to help you with chores or other responsibilities.

- Help your friend or family member learn to use public transportation.

- Talk directly to your friend or family member about his or her experiences and feelings about low vision.

- Help your friend or family member design their own exercise program and exercise regularly.

- If you have a computer, consider reprinting your friend or family member's recipes or addresses in large type and collecting them in a binder, or have them bound at a copy shop.

14. Help Start a Support Group

Support groups are a fantastic way to build community. At a low vision support group, your friend or family member would have the chance to talk to people who have walked a mile in their shoes and can understand their experience. Support groups are great places to vent, to laugh, to get new solutions for daily challenges and new ideas for living. They can also be very helpful for spouses of people with low vision. It's very comforting to talk to the "natives," as Bernie Siegel in his tape "Healing from the Inside Out," calls anyone who shares a common experience with you. If there is no support group in your area, that doesn't mean there aren't any other people with low vision. It just means that no one is getting the benefit of a support group. Why not help start one? See Chapter 6 for guidelines.

15. Keep Your Sense of Humor

We are all prone to taking life too seriously. Very few people get to the end of their lives wishing they had been more earnest, more worried, or more self-conscious. We all try so hard to get it right the first time, to avoid misfortune and mistakes, to look good in public. Sometimes we forget to laugh. Laugh from your belly, and let your friend or family member see the daily humor in this busy, unpredictable, ridiculous, profound, heartbreaking, and heartwarming experience we call living.

CHAPTER 8

I See Purple Flowers Everywhere: The Many Visions of Charles Bonnet Syndrome

"Do you ever see anything you know is not there, but looks real anyway?" I asked Sam Weinberg when he came to the Low Vision Living Program.

"No," he said, looking at his wife, Rachel, and fidgeting with his sweater.

"Oh," I said casually, "I just asked because many people with macular degeneration see things they know are not there. I call it phantom vision, but the technical term is Charles Bonnet Syndrome."

"Is this syndrome an early sign of Alzheimer's?" Sam asked pointedly, still looking at Rachel. Rachel began to look at the clock on the wall. They had been in our office for nearly two hours and Rachel felt it was already past lunch time. She picked up her coat.

"Absolutely not," I said firmly. "Charles Bonnet

Syndrome has nothing to do with mental agility or stability. When you have phantom vision, your mind is fine, it's your eyes that are playing tricks on you. It's a side effect of low vision."

"Well," Sam admitted quickly, "I see little monkeys with red hats and blue coats playing in the front yard. I've seen them for eighteen months."

"*What?*" Rachel's eyes about popped out of her head, and she dropped her coat. "*Little monkeys in the front yard?*"

"Well . . . um," Sam continued, "sometimes I see them in the living room, too."

What Is Charles Bonnet Syndrome?

Charles Bonnet was an eighteenth-century Swiss naturalist and philosopher whose grandfather, Charles Lullin, had low vision from cataracts. In 1769, Bonnet described his grandfather's curious experience of seeing men, women, birds, and buildings that he knew were not there. Later in his life, Bonnet's own vision also deteriorated and he, too, experienced phantom visions similar to his grandfather's. How could this happen? Curiously, Charles Bonnet's discovery didn't capture medical attention at the time. But 150 years later, in the 1930s, his files were dusted off, and he was credited with being the first person to describe the syndrome that came to be named for him. The medical origins of Charles Bonnet Syndrome, however, remained unclear.

Today, there are several suggested causes. The most convincing holds that the syndrome is analogous to phantom limb phenomena. People who have a limb amputated may still feel their toes or fingers, or itching on an arm that no longer exists. This happens because the limb's nerves are still active, spontaneously firing signals to the brain, which the brain dutifully interprets. So, too, with the eyes. When retinal cells become impaired, and are no longer able to receive and relay visual images to the brain, or when any other element of the visual system ceases to function optimally, the system begins firing off images on its own.

The funny thing about these images is that they are often not related to a person's life at all. Sam's monkeys, for example, were entirely original creations. He couldn't remember ever seeing these monkeys before, and he wasn't a particular fan of monkeys anyway. He found them surprising at first, especially since they seemed so vivid and lifelike, but after a while they became amusing. Since they were so clearly not real monkeys, Sam wasn't too worried about his own mind, but he was afraid that others would be, especially Rachel.

How Common Is Charles Bonnet Syndrome?

This syndrome is very common. Studies place the number somewhere between 10 percent and 40 percent of people with low vision. Twenty percent of my low vision patients have Charles Bonnet Syndrome. My research suggests that it is more likely to appear if you have a visual acuity between 20/120 and 20/400 (see Chapter 1 for an explanation of the 20/20 visual acuity measurement scale). This may be because eyes with a visual acuity between these two measurements still have a great deal of power, but aren't receiving or relaying as many images from the world as they used to. As a result, they may be adding some images of their own. We have no reliable way to know ahead of time whether you will see images, how frequently these images will occur, or how long they will last. You may never experience Charles Bonnet Syndrome, you may have it for only a few months, or you may have it for years. You may see images only a few times a month, a few times a week for a few minutes, or you may see images every day.

Are You Sure This Has Nothing to Do with Psychiatry?

Yes, phantom vision, or Charles Bonnet Syndrome, is properly a side effect of vision loss only.

Unfortunately, since ophthalmologists have rarely investigated this syndrome in the twentieth century, some psychiatric studies have used the term to describe people with visual hallucinations, people with normal vision who see things they believe are actually real. To set the record straight, I'd like to return to the six criteria for Charles Bonnet Syndrome outlined by Naville in 1873. You can use them to determine whether or not you are experiencing phantom vision. Do the images that appear to you have the following six characteristics?

- They occur when you are fully conscious and wide awake, often during broad daylight.

- They do not deceive you; you are aware that they are not real.

- They occur in combination with normal perception. For example, you may see a sidewalk clearly, but find it covered with dots, flowers, or faces.

- They are exclusively visual and do not appear in combination with any sounds or bizarre sensations.

- They appear and disappear without obvious cause.

- They are amusing or annoying, but not grotesque.

Since ophthalmology has paid so little attention to Charles Bonnet Syndrome, many doctors don't realize how common it really is, and some may not be familiar with it at all. When I gave a poster presentation of the drawings in this chapter at the American Academy of Ophthalmology's Annual Meeting in the fall of 1997, several ophthalmologists stopped to express their surprise at hearing about phantom vision for the first time.

What Do People with Charles Bonnet Syndrome See?

A 1994 Dutch study of Charles Bonnet Syndrome listed the following images seen by participants: miniature chimney sweepers, farmers, strolling children, teddy bears, windmills, chairs, women in woolly hats, and men in striped pajamas. My patients at Low Vision Living have reported seeing cartoon characters, flowers in the bathroom sink, hands rubbing one another, waterfalls and mountains, tigers, maple trees in vibrant autumn foliage, yellow polka dots, row houses, a dinner party, and brightly colored balloons. Many people see faces or life-size figures whom they've never seen before. One of the most remarkable qualities of these figures is that they almost always wear pleasant expressions and often make eye contact with the viewer. Menacing behavior, grotesque shapes, or scenes of violent conflict are not, to my knowledge, a part of this syndrome.

Usually the same image, or set of images, reappears to each person, sometimes in the same places or at the same time of day. Sam's monkeys usually materialized around sunset, cavorting across the lawn or around the big blue easy chair by the fireplace. They stayed for ten or twenty minutes several times a week for two years, and then began to appear less frequently. Sometimes the images change or multiple images appear. While Sam saw only monkeys, Joe Toscano saw chestnut horses and small rabbits on the kitchen walls. They were soon replaced by willow trees at a riverbank. Sometimes the images are exactly to scale, and sometimes larger or smaller than life. Sometimes the images become smaller the farther away they appear, and sometimes they become larger. Joe's horses looked like children's toys at a distance of ten feet, but as they galloped outside they became Clydesdales, and then stallions worthy of Gulliver.

Treating Charles Bonnet Syndrome

Fortunately, most people find Charles Bonnet Syndrome largely untroubling. Since the images it produces are usually pretty or lighthearted, many actually find them amusing or enjoyable. If, however, you find yourself frustrated or anxious, do not hesitate to discuss phantom visions with your doctor. Although no drug treatment has been demonstrated to work for everyone, the best option appears to be low dose Haldol. Usually explanation and reassurance are sufficient.

Sometimes Charles Bonnet Syndrome images can become confused with dream images. For example, several of my patients have reported frightening moments when they thought they saw a man standing in their bedroom or hallway. These men, however, were often dark-clad or indistinct figures that appeared as the patient was relaxing on a couch, dozing, or was in bed waiting to fall asleep or just awaking. These figures were probably residual dream images that reflect very normal fears of crime or loneliness. They are not, however, typical of Charles Bonnet Syndrome. As Zelda Grant put it, "Shadowy men in my bedroom? Don't be ridiculous! I see fully dressed Canadian Mounties in my bedroom with long gold sabers, big gold buttons, and stiff-brimmed blue hats. They have nice wide shoulders. They're a good-looking group."

A CHARLES BONNET PORTRAIT GALLERY

When Grace Olsen came to Low Vision Living, I asked her the same question I asked Sam Weinberg. "Do you ever see anything unusual, anything you know is not there, but appears nevertheless?" She eyed me dryly.

"Yes," she said, with an air of great patience, "but my problem is that I can't see things that *are* there. I do not much care if the kitchen sink is full of American flags. I would like to know how I can see my granddaughter's photo."

Touché! Grace was right, of course, but she was also surprised and comforted to hear that other people with low vision saw things in their sinks, too. Like Sam and Rachel Weinberg, Grace had never heard of Charles Bonnet Syndrome before; she supposed she might be the only one, so she had never shared the images she saw.

After I opened a set of felt-tip markers, we spent some time together talking about low vision and about the extraordinary set of flags, plaids, and bars of music Grace saw everywhere. The vivid colors Grace used to draw her patterns helped me understand her experience in greater detail. As she drew, Grace talked about her years as a young documentary artist for the Works Progress Administration during the Depression, and her love of all things blue: irises, jays, and oceans. Her words made me wonder anew at what a strange and stunning gift sight really is: what things we have seen, what things we remember, and what things we never expected to see. Since Grace left her drawings with me, I've asked other people with macular degeneration to depict the images they see, and to talk about their experience with Charles Bonnet Syndrome. I'd like to share their drawings and words with you.

Grace Olsen's Turquoise Squares and Bars of Music

I was in the hospital a few years ago for pneumonia. I remember sitting in my bed, waiting for lunch, when I saw light turquoise and lime green squares on the ceiling. *That's strange,* I thought, but I wasn't feeling well, so I just closed my eyes. A few weeks later, I was mixing salad dressing in the kitchen, and the same checkered pattern reappeared on the floor. Now I see it everywhere. Sometimes it's quite small, a few inches at most, and sometimes it covers a whole bedspread. I can't remember ever seeing these squares in my life. I thought they might be from one of my drawings or photographs, but I never drew abstract patterns, and my photographs were always black and white. Then I thought they came from a quilt. I used to quilt with a group, and often toured antique shops. But the lime green in this check is too rich, too goldish or brownish tinted, more like an abstract painting than a color of thread. After I became quite used to the checks, I began to see an ornate bar of music. *Good grief!* That's all I could think. I spent my childhood praying that my mother would

Grace Olsen's bars of music.

let me give up the piano. I hated
practicing so much. Why in the world
would I see a bar of music? I have tried
to read the music I see, but it doesn't
seem to play a particular tune. Just
shapes, decorative shapes.

Zelda Grant's Red Brick Building

When I was a child in North Carolina
during the Depression, I had a very old
maiden aunt, Isabel. I thought she didn't
have much fun because she never ate
cake when she came to our house. She
lived in a red brick home for the elderly.
I believed that if you didn't have any
money they sent you there. I remember
my parents whispering to one another
about money and debts. I would listen at
the door and wonder if we were all going
to live with Isabel, and if we would be
able to eat any more cake. When I saw

217

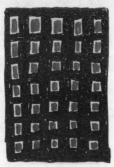

Zelda Grant's red brick building.

the red brick building, I thought of Isabel. I first saw it in the spring when my daughter and I were driving to Wilmington. I didn't mention it at first, because it looked like a classic Southern building. But then it reappeared in the next town, and the next day. I saw it all along the highway. At first I was worried. Not too worried, though, because I knew it really wasn't there. I just wasn't sure why I saw it so clearly. Then it began to amuse me. I would look for it tucked beyond a farm or a row of Main Street shops. Honestly, it's very pretty, very graceful architecturally. The landscape would be much improved if they built a few of them. I saw it for six or eight months, but I haven't seen it in a while.

Rosa Garcia's flowering trees.

Rosa Garcia's Flowering Trees

They are beautiful, these flowers. Large
vibrant pink blooms, decorating trees
with no leaves, as if flowers always grew
in the wintertime. When I first saw them,
I loved them. *This isn't possible!* I
thought. It was autumn, there were
leaves on the ground. We were on the
train to Toronto. I watched these flowers
for awhile, then I turned to my friend
Barbara and told her what I was seeing. I
remember being quite enthusiastic,
although I wasn't sure I should be saying
so much. She just sort of stared at me.
Then I made the mistake of telling her
about the chain-link fences. I had been
seeing these chain-link fences

everywhere. Well, many places they shouldn't be. They were okay. But the pink flowers were beautiful. Barbara just stared at me even harder. Then she asked a few questions about how long I had been seeing fences and flowers, and where they appeared. She didn't seem any more comfortable with my answers. For some reason, though, I didn't really care. I just stopped telling people about them. You have to be careful what you say.

Buddy Burmester's Purple Flowers and Blackbirds

I see purple flowers in my bathroom sink, and sometimes on my pants, which is a little compromising. Since no one

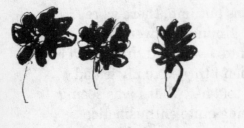

Buddy Burmester's purple flowers.

else sees them, though, I'm not so embarrassed. But can you imagine golf pants with purple flowers? I'd look like one of those hippies! I also see blackbirds. Powerful things, flying in sets of threes. My cousin Harry has macular degeneration, too. He sees frogs in his bathtub and a pretty blond woman standing on his back porch, which is very funny. Harry was never a very successful ladies' man. My purple flowers and blackbirds are not half as interesting as frogs in the bathtub and a woman on the back porch! I said to him, "Harry, maybe she's a Radio City Music Hall Rockette who made a detour through New Jersey."

"Could be," he says. "She looks like a Rockette is supposed to look. Too bad she's not really there." You ought to talk to Harry. He's not too unhappy about the whole thing.

Mary Flannery and Dolly Kowalski both saw figures of people. Although they could not draw them accurately enough to convey the tangible reality with which they originally appeared, I've included their descriptions because the figures are so representative of Charles Bonnet Syndrome.

Mary Flannery's Elizabethan Dinner Party

I was born in Belfast in 1928. My parents died just before the war, so I went to live in Boston with my Uncle Liam. My mother, of course, never liked the British. But I always loved the theater and I loved Shakespeare. I used to dress up in my aunt's old dresses and pretend I was Juliet and Romeo was on his way over to the house. I don't think that has anything to do with my Elizabethan dinner party, though. That's what I call it. I see these very formal, earnest people sitting around my dining room table in full Elizabethan dress. Their outfits are made of bright, jeweled fabrics, with lots of lace, high collars, and pinched V-shaped waists. They look like they belong on stage or in the queen's court. They're not talkative, they don't seem hungry, and they don't seem upset. Actually, they appear to think it's perfectly natural to sit around my dining room table. They irritate me sometimes, but I think my mother would probably roll over in her grave.

Dolly Kowalski's Little Girls with Pink Bows

I see little girls with pink bows playing in my yard. At first, there was only one little girl. But after a while, she had several playmates. Now they come almost every evening for fifteen minutes or so and play with one another. They laugh and jump around. They are so delightful, so cheerful, so active. Their little white dresses and pink bows blow in the wind. I see them so incredibly clearly, much more clearly than I see anything else now. I enjoy seeing the details of their dresses and the expressions on their faces. I know that they aren't real, but you wouldn't believe how realistic they seem, how lively and pretty they are. I wish you could see them the way I do.

PART III:

Visual Rehabilitation

CHAPTER 9

Starting Your Visual Rehabilitation Program

You must do the thing you think you cannot do.
—Eleanor Roosevelt

When we begin to take our failures non-seriously, it means we are ceasing to be afraid of them. It is of immense importance to learn to laugh at ourselves.
—Katherine Mansfield

Visual rehabilitation is just like rehabilitation for any other kind of impairment. If you suffer a minor stroke that impairs the use of your right arm, you will receive occupational therapy. You'll be trained to do all the daily activities you need to do without relying heavily on that arm. Low vision affects at least as many daily activities as the loss of your right arm, so visual rehabilitation provides comparable training. Visual rehabilitation includes training in using your peripheral vision to read, and training for daily activities. Visual rehabilitation also includes adapting your home with lighting, labels, and low vision products. And it includes professional fitting for magnifiers and high-power lenses, and training in their use. Some low vision programs also provide counseling and support groups.

Visual Rehabilitation Is Not Resignation

Sometimes people fear that if they pursue visual rehabilitation, they're resigning themselves to low vision, giving up on a possible cure, and giving up on their future. But visual rehabilitation is not about resignation. It's about figuring out what you would enjoy doing, pursuing it with whatever means are available, learning new skills, and letting self-judgment go. It's about having choices and influencing your life today. It's not about precluding choices that may be available tomorrow. Anyone pursuing visual rehabilitation can tell you that it doesn't foster resignation—far from it. Visual rehabilitation at its best fosters courage— the courage to try new things and keep your sense of humor. It fosters commitment—the willingness to stick with it and do the most you can. And visual rehabilitation fosters confidence—the belief that you can do more than you think you can. Right here, right now. And you can!

Finding a Visual Rehabilitation Program in Your Area

To find a visual rehabilitation program in your area, ask your doctor for a referral. You can also call the national organizations listed at the end of this book, all of which should provide program information over the phone or in print. Many states have excellent visual rehabilitation programs that are administered by the States' Commission or Agency for the Blind, although they may not accept people who have better than 20/200 vision.

There are many optometrists and some ophthalmologists who specialize in low vision, and some who offer low vision services within their regular practices. The need for visual rehabilitation has grown so quickly, however, that in some areas there are no programs easily accessible to people with low vision. If you do not have a program in your area, the Rehabilitation Workshop in this book is designed for you. It is a special home version of our Low Vision Living Program here in Michigan. You can also use this book as a supplement to your local program.

The Low Vision Living Rehabilitation Program

This rehabilitation program includes five chapters, each covering a different topic: reading with low vision, lighting, magnifiers, adapting your home, and interacting with the community. Although each chapter can be understood independently, the chapters were written to build upon one another. As a result, each chapter assumes that you know the information covered in the previous one. For example, Chapter 13, which talks about adaptations you can make to your home, assumes that you already know about the lighting information covered in Chapter 11 and the magnifier information covered in Chapter 12. For this reason, it's best to proceed through each chapter in the order in which they are presented.

This is particularly true for Chapter 10, Your Reading Workshop, which must be followed exactly as presented. The entire workshop, including the complete reading practice program, will take an hour or so a day for two to four weeks. You may choose to begin the Reading Workshop now and read the other chapters while you complete the workshop, or you may choose to read the other chapters first and begin the workshop afterward.

You may find all of the information in this section easy to digest and you may want to read or listen quickly. On the other hand, many people find it much easier to take one chapter at a time at their own pace, especially since most of the chapters give a lot of advice for changing things in your home, learning new skills, or using new products. You may also want to order the free low vision product catalogs listed in the appendix and browse through them as you work through the program.

WORKING WITH A FAMILY MEMBER OR FRIEND

Most of Low Vision Living's Rehabilitation Program does not directly call for assistance from friends or family members. The Reading Workshop is an exception. You will need a partner for the first exercise, and you may find that working with someone for the second exercise will help a great deal. However, the whole program does implicitly assume that you have a friend or family member at hand. Obviously, if you have macular degeneration you may not be able to read regular size print. Even if you can read this book or are listening on tape, you may find that you'd like help with certain projects or new skills like re-arranging your furniture, browsing through low vision product catalogs, or learning to use the subway system. Working with friends or family members on visual rehabilitation can also make the program more enjoyable. And they'll learn a lot, too. In fact, there are several tips for friends and family along the way.

Arranging Assistance

You may want to skim through the whole program first with a friend or family member to determine which parts you already know, which you may be able to do on your own or with minimal assistance, and which parts will take more time. The amount of assistance you may need and the pace at which you work through the program will vary depending upon your own circumstances and preferences. You may already have one family member or friend who can serve as a partner for the whole program. If not, consider asking several friends or family members to each help with a portion. To accommodate everyone's schedules, consider setting up appointments in advance for reading chapters or working on rehabilitation tasks or tips. This approach may be particularly helpful for the Reading Workshop.

SUPPLIES TO PURCHASE OR HAVE HANDY

Chapter 10, Your Reading Workshop, and Chapter 13, Saving Sight in Your Home, both call for a small collection of inexpensive supplies. You can find almost everything on both of these lists at a local office supply store. You may want to collect them before you begin your rehabilitation program.

SUPPLIES FOR CHAPTER 10, YOUR READING WORKSHOP

- 1 thick black felt-tip pen
- 1 package of at least sixty plain white three-by-five-inch index cards

- 1 package of ready-made stick-on (sticky) black letters one to one-and-a-half inches high. Sticky letters are available at most office supply shops. If you cannot find them, you can use your black felt-tip marking pen to print individual letters.

To do the Reading Workshop, you will need a table or desk with strong glare-free light directed onto the reading material. Overhead lighting or light from a regular shade lamp may not be sufficient. You may want to purchase or borrow a small, inexpensive gooseneck table lamp with an indoor incandescent floodlight bulb.

SUPPLIES FOR CHAPTER 13, SAVING SIGHT IN YOUR HOME

- 1 medium width black permanent marker

- 1 package of large rubber bands
(continued)

- 1 small package of safety pins

- Large black, white, and bright neon orange stickers

- Ready-made stick-on (sticky) black letters one to two inches high, or higher if they are more easily readable

- 1 tube each of black, white, and orange puff paint. Puff paint is available at many fabric stores and is sometimes marketed as fabric or T-shirt paint. You can squeeze it onto fabric, metal, or other surfaces for labeling. Since it dries slightly puffy, you can also feel it.

SUPPLIES TO GATHER FOR YOURSELF

Now that you are starting your visual rehabilitation program and purchasing the supplies you need for various chapters, don't forget the most important supplies of all: the ones you need for you. Visual rehabilitation can make living easier, but it does take some determination and courage. And like all things worth having in life, it takes some work and some humor, too. You've got all the skills and qualities you'll need—but gathering them together as you start your program and keeping them at your fingertips will help you have a positive, empowering experience. Remember, you do have choices. You can influence the quality of your life. Beginning a visual rehabilitation program, and committing to living fully in the world in whatever way is best for you, are choices. It is a choice to positively influence the quality of your life. You can do it. I know you can.

SUPPLIES FOR YOU: THE THREE C'S

- **Courage:** trying new things and keeping your sense of humor

- **Commitment:** sticking with it and doing the most you can

- **Confidence:** believing you can do more than you think you can

---

Your Reading Workshop

That which we persist in doing becomes easier to do, not that the nature of the task has changed, but our ability to do it has increased.
—Ralph Waldo Emerson

We often think of reading as a skill that we learned years ago in grade school. Now we simply know how to read. But reading is actually more like playing tennis: it's very practice sensitive. Just as your tennis game improves with practice, so your reading ability improves with practice, too. As a rule, the more we read, the more efficiently we can read. This is true of everyone, especially everyone with low vision. And it's true of all kinds of reading, not just reading novels or articles, but reading signs and labels, too. If you haven't been reading for a while because of low vision, you may not be able to read as much as you actually could with training and practice. The Reading Workshop will teach you new techniques for reading with low vision and help you practice them. Even if you aren't interested in reading, reading practice is still the best way to learn how to maximize your sight in other situations. Reading practice will make it easier to identify packages in the grocery store, see food at the table, crochet, or walk down the sidewalk, because reading practice trains you to use the clearest areas of your remaining vision most effectively.

Magnifiers and the Reading Workshop

There is another great reason to complete the Reading Workshop: many people find that it enables them to use weaker magnifiers, sometimes magnifiers as much as two or three times (X powers) weaker. This is good because weaker magnifiers are usually easier to use than stronger ones. They cover a wider area of print, and you can hold them farther from your eyes, so they give you a more comfortable reading distance.

Lighting and the Reading Workshop

Really good lighting is absolutely necessary for the Reading Workshop. In fact, good lighting is necessary whenever you read. You will not be able to do the exercises in this chapter without good lighting. I recommend a gooseneck or adjustable table or floor lamp with an indoor floodlight bulb. Adjust the lamp so it shines directly on the exercise or reading material. Do not use a regular incandescent light bulb that is less than 100 watts or lamps with regular shades that do not shine light directly on the material. Overhead lighting, no matter how bright, may not be sufficient, especially if you lean over while you read, casting shadows on the material.

Inside Your Reading Workshop

Anne T. Riddering, M.A., O.T.R. is the director of occupational therapy at our visual rehabilitation program in Michigan. We all call her Annie. She designed this Reading Workshop especially for you to use at home. It's almost the same one she does here with our patients. The workshop has three exercises. You must complete all three exercises in the order in which they appear.

The first exercise, "Finding Your Scotoma," takes about an hour. Annie usually does this exercise with our patients in their homes. You will need an "Annie," too: a friend or family member who can work with you. In this exercise you will find the weakest area of your central vision and practice moving it out of the way in order to see clearly.

The second exercise, "Relearning to Read," may take anywhere from a few hours to several days. In this exercise you will relearn which letters of the alphabet look alike, making it easier for you to quickly identify a misleading letter when you encounter it. Annie spends time with our patients on this one, too—so you may want your friend or family member to help.

The third exercise, "Reading Practice," is an extended reading practice program you can do on your own that will take one hour a day for two to four weeks.

Confidence, Commitment, and Courage

Ah! you may be thinking, *this is going to take some effort.* And you're right. It will. But it'll be worth the effort. You may find the workshop enjoyable and fairly easy. Or you may find it challenging. But you can do it, and it will help you to read print and to see just about anything else more effectively. Gather your confidence, courage, and commitment, and set them next to you. Be determined, but be kind to yourself, too. Stick with the exercises. Take breaks when you're tired or frustrated. Be sure to give yourself rewards for trying. If you have a hard time working alone, ask someone to do the workshop with you. And don't worry about your pace. Remember, it was the tortoise who won the race in Aesop's fable, not the hare. You can do it. Go for it!

DO NOT USE MAGNIFIERS FOR THE READING WORKSHOP

Do not use your magnifiers for any part of the Reading Workshop, including "Reading Practice." Wear your regular reading glasses or no glasses at all if you read better without them. Magnifiers come later, in Chapter 12.

GETTING STARTED: WORKSHOP MATERIALS.

Collect the following materials:

- 1 "Annie" (family member or friend who can be your partner for the first exercise, and perhaps the second, too). Read through this chapter with your partner to get a sense of how much time you may need together.

- 1 package of fifty-two plain, unlined white three-by-five-inch index cards.

- 1 package of ready-made stick-on black letters one to one-and-a-half inches high.

Make sure you have the entire alphabet in both capital and lower case letters. You can find stick-on letters at many office supply stores, drugstores, superstores, and low vision catalogs. If these letters are not available, you can use a thick black felt-tip marker to print your own.

Preparing the Materials

Place one ready-made stick-on letter lengthwise at the top of each index card—the top of the letter should be pointing toward the short side of the index card—so you have the entire alphabet in both capital and lower case letters, with only one letter on each card. If you are using a felt-tip marker, write one letter at the top of each index card in capitals and again in lower case letters until you have the whole alphabet in each case, with only one letter on each card. Try to make your letters very clear and even, and one to one-and-a-half inches high. You will need these cards to find your scotoma and to retrain your eyes to recognize letters with low vision.

EXERCISE 1: FINDING YOUR SCOTOMA

The first goal of the Reading Workshop is to find your scotoma. Your scotoma is the area of your central vision with the lowest acuity, in other

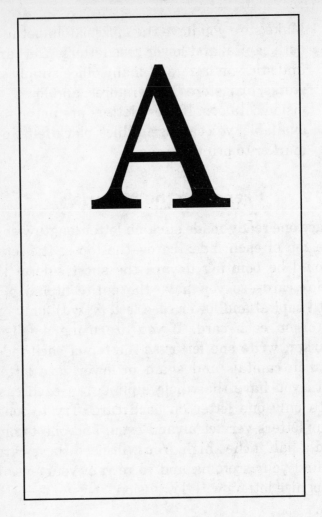

words the area that gives you the blurriest picture. You might wonder why we should look for
this area, rather than the area that sees the
clearest. The answer is that you probably already

know which area of your central vision sees the clearest, even if you aren't aware that you know. Most people automatically adjust to low vision by moving their eyes when they look at an object so they can see it with the area of their central vision that provides the clearest view. However, most people are not aware of which area (or areas) provide the blurriest view. If you know which area provides the blurriest view, and you learn to move it out of the way, you will have covered both of your bases. You'll naturally look at things with the best area of your vision. And if that doesn't automatically work, you'll also know how to move the worst part of your vision out of the way in order to produce the clearest view.

Ring Scotomas and Multiple Scotomas

Most people's scotoma is close to the center of their vision, so that the clearest areas of their vision will be farther out around the edges. You may have only one scotoma, especially if you have relatively good vision, although some people have more than one. If you have multiple scotomas, focus on finding the blurriest one. About 20 percent of people with macular degeneration have a ring scotoma, which is a scotoma that forms a ring around your central vision, leaving a small, clearer area in the middle. This means that you may see things fairly clearly, but you also may lose the image quickly if you move your eye slightly. If you have a ring scotoma, practicing keeping your eye directly on whatever you wish to see, and moving your scotoma out of the way when necessary, will be very helpful.

Finding Your Scotoma

Our natural instinct is to move our eyes toward any object we want to see. To find your scotoma, however, you must keep your eyes on your partner's nose throughout the exercise. Read all seven steps first so you understand the whole exercise, and then begin with the first.

Step 1

Position two chairs facing each other so that their seats are a foot or so apart. Hardback or kitchen chairs may be easiest to maneuver. Sit facing your partner so your knees are nearly touching. Don't wear your glasses, unless you absolutely cannot do the exercise without them. Do not use any magnifiers.

Step 2

Look at your partner's nose. If you cannot see his or her nose, look directly at the spot where you know the nose should be. Do not move your eyes during the exercise. Your partner should watch your eyes to make sure you are always looking at his or her nose.

Step 3

Your partner selects a card with a capital letter and holds the card up facing you, so that it is halfway between the two of you, at the same height as the top of your forehead. If your face were a clock, your partner would be holding the card at twelve o'clock.

Step 4

Try to identify the letter.

Step 5

Your partner selects another card and holds it in the one o'clock position. Try to identify this new letter. Continue around all twelve points of the clock, with a new letter for each point. Finally, your partner selects yet another letter and places it in the center of the clock, moving it a few inches up, down, to the right, and to the left. Identify the letter.

Step 6

As you go around the clock, you and your partner should notice the position in which the letter is hardest to identify or disappears altogether. This is where your scotoma is.

Step 7

Confirm and remember the location of your scotoma by double-checking it. Your partner selects another letter and holds it where you can see it, then moves it into your scotoma so that it

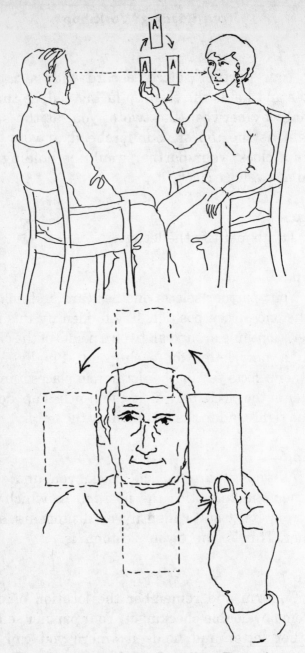

Illustrations of the Reading Exercise.

disappears or becomes blurry. Repeat this until you are sure you know where it is.

What If I Don't Find my Scotoma?

If you don't find your scotoma, don't worry, especially if you know you have pretty good vision. Your scotoma is probably very small. On the other hand, you may want to double-check the following possibilities and try the exercise again:

- Make sure you are looking at your partner's nose at all times. You may be moving your eyes to avoid your scotoma when you look at the letter.

- Make sure you aren't reading the letter before your partner puts it in a test position. Sometimes, if you already know what the letter is, your brain will automatically fill in the image, making it look clearer than it is.

- Use lower case letters, smaller sticky letters, or print smaller letters on additional index cards and use them instead. Capital letters may be too large to catch your scotoma.

What if my Scotoma Seems to Be Everywhere?

If your scotoma seems to be everywhere, double-check the following possibilities and try the exercise again:

- You may not have enough well-directed light in the room. Add lighting or move to a brighter area.

- Your partner may be holding the card too far out to the side or too close to his or her own nose. Have your partner adjust his or her placement of the card.

- The letters on the card may be too small for you to read. Print a larger letter on a card with a thick black marker. Repeat the exercise using the larger letter.

If your scotoma still seems to be everywhere, and you have moderate to very low vision (20/150 or higher), you may have a complicated scotoma pattern. Ideally, you should go to a low vision rehabilitation program with a scanning laser ophthalmoscope (SLO). The SLO can photograph your scotoma pattern so your doctor knows exactly where your best areas of vision are. You can call the national organizations listed in the back of the book for references, or ask your doctor for a referral. If the program you find does not have an SLO, go anyway. They will be able to help you find your scotoma and fit you correctly with magnifiers, as well as provide training in their use. If you can't find a program, don't worry. You can still benefit from the rest of the Reading Workshop.

Practice Moving Your Scotoma

You can move your scotoma out of the way by moving your eye toward it. This may seem counter-intuitive at first, but try it until you're comfortable. Whenever you are reading and you have particular trouble, try moving your scotoma out of the way by moving your eye toward it. This may take some practice, which you can do along with exercises 2 and 3, but once you can do so easily, it will help your reading a great deal.

EXERCISE 2: RELEARNING TO READ

When we learned to read in grade school we had to memorize each letter of the alphabet. It was a challenging task at the time because the letters look a lot alike. By now, though, we're so used to them that we don't realize how confusing they can be. More importantly, we don't realize that they are confusing in a predictable way. Since certain letters look alike, we will almost always confuse them with each other, rather than with letters that look significantly different. In order to read efficiently with low vision, you need to relearn what you first learned in grade school: which letters you are likely to confuse. When you have this information at your fingertips, you can quickly double-check a letter by considering the logical alternatives.

Don't be discouraged by the number of letters involved in this exercise. Make a game of it; take them one group at a time. Everyone has difficulties remembering them at first but you can do it! It just takes patience and practice.

Relearning Capital Letters

Begin with the capital letters and do not continue to the lower case letters until you feel confident that you have memorized the capitals. Trying to do too many letters at once can be overwhelming. Go through all five steps without worrying about remembering every letter the first time around. This will give you an understanding of the whole exercise. Once you have gone through all five steps, return to the first step and begin again. This time, try to memorize the letter groups. Test yourself with your index cards once a day until you know the letter groups by heart. Notice which letters are most confusing to you, and pay special attention to them.

Step 1: The Two X's

Take out your **X** and **K** and put them on the table next to each other. Now cover the left side of each letter and you will see that the right sides are almost identical. So when you see what you think is either an **X** or a **K**, be sure to double-check the left side of the letter to tell the difference.

Step 2: The Four Straight Arrows

Take out **I, T, J,** and **L** and put them on the table next to each other. Their straight lines make them look very similar, especially if the font in which they are printed doesn't exaggerate their differences.

Step 3: The Four Round Ones

Take out your **C, G, O,** and **Q** and put them on the table next to each other. Notice that they all share identical left sides. If you cover the right side of each letter, they look the same. So when you see one of these four letters, remember to double-check the right side of the letter to tell the differences.

And Their Flat-Sided Cousins

Leave the **O** on the table and put **D** and **U** next to it. Notice that if the tops were gone, they look almost like triplets. If you think you see one of these three letters, double-check the top of the letter to tell the difference.

Step 4: The Five Straight-Round Combos

Take out **E** and **F** and put them next to each other. Then take out **B, P,** and **R** and put them next to each other. Cover the bottom right corner of **E** and **F** and you'll see that they look alike. Then cover the bottom right corner of **B, P,** and **R** and they'll look the same, too. **B** can also sometimes look like **S**. Now cover the right side of **F, P,** and **R** and they'll look alike.

Step 5: The Five Diagonal Devils

These letters are the toughest of all. Take out the **N, M, W, V,** and **Y** and put them next to each other. You will see that they are all combinations of straight and diagonal lines, which can be very confusing. To tell them apart, look carefully at the bottoms of the letters.

REVIEWING AND REMEMBERING CAPITAL LETTERS

The two X's:	X, K
The Four Straight Arrows:	I, T, J, L
The Four Round Ones:	C, G, O, Q
Their Flat-Sided Cousins:	D, U
The Five Straight-Round Combos:	E, F, B, P, R
The Five Diagonal Devils:	N, M, W, V, Y

Congratulations!
You're halfway there.
Don't give up!

Relearning Lower Case Letters

Step 1: Dots and Crosses, and the L

Take out the **l, i,** and **j.** To tell them apart, you need to look at the top of the letter to see if there is a dot, and the bottom to see whether or not the letter is an **i** or a **j.** Now leave the **l** on the table, and place it next to the **t** and **f.** As with the dots, you need to look at the top of the letter to double-check the cross and then see if there is a curl indicating an **f.** Of course, if there is no dot and no cross, you always have an **l.**

Step 2: The Little Round Vowels

Take out the **c, e, o** and **a** (some forms of **a** are entirely round, resembling an **o**). To tell these letters apart, you need to look at their right sides.

Step 3: One Hump or Two, or Is It a U?

Take out **m, n,** and **u.** These three are nearly identical triplets when they're buried in the middle of a word. You can tell them apart if you make a point of looking at the top of the letter where you can see if it's open or closed and how many humps it has.

Step 4: The Pot Bellies and Straight Backs

Take out the **b, d, h,** and **p** and set them next to one another. These are the pot bellies and straight backs. They can be confusing because they all have a stem and some form of roundness that may be open or closed at the bottom. When you come across any of these letters, be sure to look first at the top and then at the bottom to double-check the stems and openings of the letters. This strategy of double-checking stems and openings will also help you with **h, n,** and **r**. In some fonts **g, q,** and **p** also look similar.

REVIEWING AND REMEMBERING THE LOWER CASE LETTERS

The Two Dots and	i, j, l and
Two Crosses:	f, t, l
The Little Round Vowels:	c, e, o, a
One Hump or Two, or Is It a U?:	m, n, u
The Pot Bellies and	b, d, h, p,
Straight Backs:	h, n, r
	and g, q, p
The Diagonal Devils Revisited:	v, w, y

Step 5: Diagonal Devils Revisited

Take out **v, w,** and **y**. These three letters are just as likely to be confused in lower case as they are in their upper case forms. To tell the difference, look at the bottom to check for the stem of the **y**, and then look at the top to check the number of points to tell if it's either a **v** or **w**.

Congratulations!
You've done it!
Great job!

EXERCISE 3: READING PRACTICE

Now you can apply the skills you've learned from exercises 1 and 2 to reading. The next few pages reprint selected passages from several books: Sarah and Elizabeth Delany's *Having Our Say, The Little Prince* by Antoine de Saint Exupéry, *Plain Speaking* by Merle Miller, and *The Old Man and the Sea* by Ernest Hemingway. Each passage is in different type size. Choose the smallest size that you can read without straining and without using a magnifier. Begin practicing with this passage. Read the passage continually for at least fifteen minutes at a time, three times a day for a week. If it becomes very easy, try the next smaller size print. Continue reading three times a day for one week and moving down to the next smaller size print when the reading becomes easy. When you have reached the smallest print size that you can read, practice for one more week.

If all six fonts are too small for you, take this book to a copy shop and ask the clerk to copy the largest passage below at 120 percent or 130 percent of its size. Check this sample to see if you can read it without straining. If you are still straining, enlarge the print even more. Continue enlarging until you find a print size you can read without straining. Keep your other copies. As you practice, you may be able to use them to move down to the next smaller size. Since it may take several tries to find a size that works for you, you may want to call the copy shop ahead of time for an appointment or arrive at the least busy time of day.

We think you will enjoy these passages but if you would like to practice with something else or you begin to memorize these, you can vary your reading by enlarging any book page or magazine article to the appropriate size. There are two excellent workbooks for readers with low vision: "Learn to Use Your Vision for Reading" (LUV Reading) by Wright and Watson and the "McGill Low Vision Manual" by Overbury and Conrad. Ordering information for both workbooks is listed in Appendix I. It doesn't matter what you read. What matters is that you read the smallest size print that you can without straining and without visual aids. If you read print that is too large and too easy to see, you won't be challenged to use your new reading skills. If you read print that is

too small, you will tire and become too frustrated
to really exercise your new skills.

From
Having Our Say

Mama was starting to shrink up and get bent
down, and I started exercising with her to
straighten her up again. Only I didn't know
at that time that what we were actually
doing was "yoga." We just thought we were
exercising.

I kept doing my yoga exercises, even after
Mama died. Well, when Bessie turned eighty
she decided that I looked better than her. So
she decided she would start doing yoga, too.
So we've been doing our exercises together
ever since. We follow a yoga exercise program
on the TV. Sometimes, Bessie cheats. I'll be
doing an exercise and look over at her, and
she's just lying there! She's a naughty old gal.

*   *   *

Sometimes, when I realize I
am 101 years old, it hits me
right between the eyes. I say,

"Oh, Lord, how did this happen?" . . .

There's a few things I have had to give up. I gave up driving a while back. I guess I was in my late eighties. That was terrible. Another thing I gave up on was cutting back my trees so we have a view of the New York city skyline to the south. Until I was ninety-eight years old, I would climb up on the ladder and saw those tree branches off so we had a view. I could do it perfectly well; why pay somebody to do it? Then Sadie talked some sense into me, and I gave up doing it.

From
Plain Speaking

We saved our dimes, threw them into the tray of an old trunk, and they accumulated faster than you'd think even in those days, and then my father sent away . . . and we got the nicest set of Shakespeare you ever did see and a book of Plutarch's *Lives*. My father used to read to me out loud from that. And I've read Plutarch through many times since . . . He knew more about politics than all the other writers I've read put together.

When I was in politics, there would be times when I tried to figure somebody out, and I could always turn to Plutarch, and nine times out of ten I'd be able to find a parallel in there . . . The only thing new in the world is the history you don't know.

From
The Old Man and the Sea

He looked down into the water and watched the lines that went straight down into the dark of the water. He kept them straighter than anyone did, so that at each level

in the darkness of
the stream there
would be bait
waiting exactly
where he wished
it to be for any
fish that swam
there. Others let
them drift with
the current and
sometimes they
were at sixty
fathoms when the

fishermen thought they were at a hundred.

But, he thought, I keep them with precision. Only I have no luck anymore. But who knows? Maybe today. Every day is a new day. It is better to be lucky. But I would rather be exact. Then when luck comes you are ready.

From
Plain Speaking

You have the best time in the world on a farm like ours. You've always got the stock to take care

of, and you've got
people coming in
to talk to you
about whether
you can help
them out in
harvesting the
wheat or plant-
ing the corn . . .
Farmers really
all have time to
think, and some
of them do it,

and those are the ones who have made it possible for us to have free government. That's what Jefferson was writing about. Farmers have more time to think than city people do.

From *The Little Prince*

"All men have the stars," he answered, "but they are not the same things for different people. For some, who are travelers, the stars are guides. For others they are no more than little lights in the sky. For others, who are scholars, they are problems. For my businessman they were wealth. But all these stars are silent. You— you alone— will have the stars as no one else has them—".

CHAPTER 11

Making Things Brighter: Lighting

Lighting goes with *everything*. Doing something? You need good light. That's the bottom line. But it's surprising how little we actually think about light, or realize that we can dramatically change the lighting in our own home. Every week Annie and I meet people who don't realize that they need more light now than they used to. "One new patient sent me back to the office when I arrived at her house for a rehabilitation appointment," Annie told me recently. "We had talked the week before over the phone, and she listened to everything I said about light. When I arrived for our appointment, she greeted me with a big smile and said, 'Annie! You're not going to believe this, but I changed every light bulb in my house and now I'm seeing things I haven't seen in a year.'" Another patient, to her amazement, found herself able to read print twice as small as she usually could by using a focused-beam halogen desk lamp. Not all problems can be solved so easily, but increasing lighting and reducing glare will help tremendously.

Reducing Glare

If you have macular degeneration, you may be sensitive to glare, especially from fluorescent lights or sunlight. This happens because macular degeneration may affect your eye's ability to modulate light. You can reduce glare by choosing softer light sources, like incandescent lights over fluorescent lights or by changing your position in relationship to the light source. For example, facing sunlight may be much less comfortable than facing away, and allowing the sunlight to fall over your shoulder or come from the side if you are using a magnifier. Shiny book pages are often much more difficult to look at than matte finished pages. The same is true of highly polished furniture and floors; they can produce glare where carpeting, secured area rugs, and upholstered furniture would not. Reducing glare is an important component of good lighting in your home. If you are extremely glare sensitive, you may choose to do some things, like dining at home or in restaurants, with less light than we recommend in this chapter. You may also choose to reduce the amount of sunlight in your home. As with every aspect of visual rehabilitation, the trick is to make the environment comfortable for you.

THE ONE-DAY OBSERVATION

You may already be aware of exactly when and where you need to add light or reduce glare in your home. But oftentimes we unconsciously adjust to low lighting without realizing that we are living with less light than we really need. Lighting conditions in our homes and our lighting needs also change depending upon the time of day and the type of activity we are pursuing. To help identify your home lighting conditions and lighting needs, take one day to observe lighting in your home by walking through it three times: once in the early morning, once in the afternoon, and once in the evening. If you live in an area with variable weather or seasons, you may want to observe your home more than once to see how changes in outdoor lighting affect your ability to see inside. Notice the following:

1. Which areas of your home have only medium or low lighting? Are your stairwells, porches, and closets adequately lit? Do you have bright, focused light in the areas where you do detailed work, like reading or cooking?

2. Which areas receive a great deal of sunlight and which do not? At which times of the day? How does your window dressing affect the amount of sunlight in your home?

3. Where does glare bother you? Is the glare from sunlight, light fixtures, or reflections?

4. During the same twelve-hour period, notice moments when you have trouble seeing. Ask yourself where you are sitting or standing when you find yourself frustrated. What are the lighting conditions?

Now that you have a more thorough understanding of the lighting conditions in your home and your particular lighting needs, you can use the information in the rest of this chapter to choose the changes that will be most effective for you.

INCREASING LIGHTING IN YOUR HOME

Lighting is very personal. What works for one person may not work for another, so you may have to experiment a bit with furniture arrangements, window dressings, fixtures, and light bulbs to find the combination that works best for you. The next few paragraphs outline lighting options. A list of the most popular suggestions for people with macular degeneration follows below.

Using Sunlight in Your Home

While you are choosing new fixtures or bulbs, or rearranging the lighting in your home, don't forget to use your free lighting—sunlight. Allow as much sunlight as you can into your home without tolerating too much glare. Sunlight is brighter and more powerful than artificial light. You can often see color contrasts or read better with sunlight than with lamps. If you do have bright afternoon light in your home, take your clothing choices for the following day to the sunniest room to make your selection, rather than choosing your clothing in the morning when your home is relatively dark. You may also want to rearrange your furniture or rooms to take advantage of the rhythms of sunlight. For example, if you like to drink coffee and do a crossword puzzle in the morning, you may be better off relaxing in a sunny bedroom than struggling to see in a sunless kitchen or living room. If you do sit in the sun, position your chair or couch with its back against the window so that the light falls on your page or coffee cup. You may also be better off replacing your heavy drapes with sheer curtains or blinds to allow as much sunlight as possible while reducing glare. Vertical blinds are an excellent option because you can track the sun all day.

Light Fixture Options

There are essentially three categories of home light fixtures: fixed overhead lighting, inflexible floor or table lamps, and flexible desk lamps (gooseneck type or hinge type).

Overhead fixtures provide basic overall room light but are generally not adequate for detailed work. Inflexible floor or table lamps are also good for overall room light but do not always provide as much light as we assume they do. They tend to throw light toward the ceiling and the floor, providing only moderate to low light at eye level. Traditional shade lamps are the worst, since the shades mute most of the light and throw the rest all over the room. If your incandescent ceiling or floor fixtures aren't adequately lighting your rooms, try using at least 100 watt bulbs. For brighter light, you may consider a halogen pedestal lamp that sits on the floor (also called a torchiere). Many people buy one for the room in which they spend the most time. Halogen lamps do have one serious drawback: they are very hot and can cause fires if they are knocked down on carpets or positioned too closely to drapes. For this reason, they are now sold with protective metal screens over the bulbs. Use them with caution.

For desk lamps, many people prefer halogen fixtures and bulbs because they are so bright. A 50 watt halogen reflector bulb gives light equivalent to a 150 watt incandescent bulb. However, some people find halogen desk lamps too hot. The most convenient fixture for detailed work is a gooseneck or hinge type adjustable table or floor lamp with an indoor floodlight bulb. They are particularly good if you are sensitive to glare, because you can position the light beam below the level of your eyes, and still direct strong illumination onto a page or project. You can adjust the brightness of desk and floor lamps by moving them farther away, choosing fixtures with dimmers, or by changing lightbulbs.

Lightbulb Options

There are four different types of lightbulbs available at hardware stores, superstores or through low vision catalogs: fluorescent, halogen, chromalux, and incandescent (incandescent bulbs come in two models: regular or floodlight). Each type has advantages and disadvantages.

Fluorescent and halogen bulbs provide the brightest light, which many people appreciate, but they do have some drawbacks. Fluorescent bulbs can only be used in fixtures designed for them; they also tend to cause glare, which can be extremely irritating. Halogen bulbs cause less glare but tend to be more expensive, and they are sometimes too bright, too hot, or too heavy for desk lamps. For these reasons, halogen bulbs are best used in pedestal floor lamps. Traditional halogen bulbs fit only in halogen lamps, but halogen reflector bulbs do have standard bases that can fit any lamp.

Chromalux and incandescent bulbs are somewhat similar. Chromalux bulbs are available in 60 and 100 watt frosted glass; they are designed to imitate natural light and are cooler than ordinary incandescent bulbs. Incandescent bulbs, which are the familiar regular light bulbs, are cheaper and more widely available. In higher wattages, however, they tend to be hot and are not quite as bright as fluorescent or halogen. For this reason, incandescent floodlight bulbs are very popular with people who have macular degeneration because they provide brighter, more focused light without adding more wattage or heat. We often find that they are the best bulbs of all.

CAUTION

When you purchase new fixtures, make sure that your electrical system can handle any extra wattage. When you use stronger bulbs in new or existing fixtures, make sure you follow the manufacturer's instructions. Using the wrong lightbulb in a fixture can ruin your fixture and short your entire electrical system.

THE MOST POPULAR SUGGESTIONS FOR INCREASING LIGHTING

- Replace your incandescent light bulbs that are less than 75 to 100 watts with 75 to 100 watt bulbs. For detailed work, use a 50 to 65 watt incandescent indoor floodlight or a halogen reflector bulb.

- Buy a small, inexpensive gooseneck or hinge type lamp with an indoor floodlight bulb. Make sure it is easy to carry and adjust. Take this lamp with you around the house to places where you most frequently need light for detailed work, like reading or setting laundry dials. Perch it on tabletops, sinks, counters, appliances, or desks. In the areas where you use it most frequently, consider purchasing one to place there permanently. You can find models for $10 to $25 at local hardware stores or superstores that sit on any surface, screw into walls, or clip onto desktops or bed frames.

- Buy a bright, lightweight flashlight or penlight. Make sure it is not too heavy. Carry it in your pocket or purse. Use it to read labels in the grocery store, menus in restaurants, or to see things around your house, like clothes in the closet, stove dials, alarm systems, thermostats, and cleaning fluid bottles in the garage. Camping stores are often the best sources for strong, lightweight flashlights.

THE MOST POPULAR SUGGESTIONS FOR REDUCING GLARE

- Replace irritating fluorescent lights with incandescent light fixtures. Use at least 75 to 100 watt incandescent bulbs, indoor floodlight bulbs, or chromalux bulbs.

- Cover Formica countertops, glass tables, or shiny polished wood tables with tablecloths or towels. Cover polished hardwood floors or tile floors that reflect glare with heavy area rugs. Make sure you secure all rugs so they do not slide and you do not trip on their edges. Move mirrors that reflect glare.

- Use venetian blinds or, better yet, sheer curtains to reduce sun glare while allowing as much sunlight as possible into your home.

- To reduce unavoidable glare in your home, grocery stores, or restaurants, wear a pair of light yellow or plum NOIR (wraparound) glasses. These glasses can be worn alone or over your prescription glasses. They are available through the low vision catalogs listed in the back of this book for $15 to $20.

- To reduce glare outside, wear a pair of blue-blocker sunglasses or add blue-blockers to your existing sunglasses or regular glasses, or wear a pair of dark yellow NOIR glasses either by themselves or over your regular glasses. Blue-blockers will increase the tint of your lenses and cut glare, but they will not decrease the overall amount of light you perceive. In other words, unlike regular sunglasses, they will not make the world look darker. Talk to your optician about these options, and see Chapter 3 for more information on blue-blockers.

LIGHTING IN PUBLIC PLACES

Unfortunately, we often get too much sunlight outside, and too little inside. Many restaurants keep their lighting low to create ambiance, while grocery stores blast fluorescent lights to highlight their products. So what can you do? Keep a pair of lightly tinted wraparound glasses with you to reduce indoor glare (see above) and carry a small flashlight or penlight for reading print or identifying objects in poorly lit stores and restaurants. When you dine out, request a table with good lighting or one near a sunny window. Sit with your back to the window so that the sunlight falls on the menu and on your plate. If you find a restaurant with particularly good lighting and a friendly staff, compliment them and give them your business.

Restaurants need to know that low lighting and fluorescent lighting can be extremely inconvenient for their customers and can discourage seniors from returning. Remember, you aren't alone. There are more than 1.5 million Americans with advanced macular degeneration who need more light to see. They like to dine out, too.

CHAPTER 12

Making Things Bigger:
Magnifiers

As we go about our daily activities, let us maintain a positive attitude, knowing full well that there are more sophisticated devices constantly being made available to us to help in daily living.

—Bert Silverman
ARMD patient
and author of
<u>Bert's Eye View:</u>
<u>Coping with Macular Degeneration</u>

Magnifiers are fantastic tools. You can do all kinds of things with magnifiers that aren't possible without them. But magnifiers are also tricky. My patients often tell me that their thoughtful son or daughter gave them a perfectly good magnifier for their birthday and it doesn't work at all. Technically, magnifiers always work. Their job is to magnify and they always do. But magnifiers are made in different strengths and styles, and they magnify clearly only when they are held at the correct distance. You have to choose magnifiers with the right strength or power for your visual acuity; you have to choose the right styles for your needs; you have to use your magnifiers correctly; and you have to have adequate lighting. Since magnifiers are rarely sold with purchasing instructions or users' manuals, it's very easy to get the wrong one if you're choosing on your own. And it's true that the wrong magnifier will not work for you.

BUYING MAGNIFIERS

More Expensive is Not Always Better

Magnifiers vary tremendously not only in strength, but in style and price. There are different kinds of magnifiers for reading, doing detailed work with both hands, distance viewing, and walking around. Magnifiers come in all shapes, sizes, and weights. They come attached to various handles, stands, headsets, neck cords, and jewelry chains. Some magnifiers require you to hold them steady, others don't. And they cost anywhere from $10 to $1,000 or more, especially if you consider lamp magnifiers, electronic magnifiers, or computer magnifying software. More expensive, however, does not always mean better. If you have pretty good vision and you want to read the newspaper, a $350 high-tech lamp magnifier will be less useful to you than an inexpensive goose-neck desk lamp with a floodlight and a $35 paper-weight magnifier. On the other hand, if you have less than 20/400 vision, the absolute best magni-fier for reading anything will be a video magni-fier, also called a closed circuit television (CCTV). The bottom line is that the right magnifier for you is the one that enables you to do exactly what you want with the greatest ease.

How Much Money Can You Expect to Spend?

You probably need at least three or four magni-fiers: a portable hand magnifier for spot reading, a stand magnifier for continuous reading, a head-mounted magnifier for doing something with both your hands, and a distance magnifier. These basic magnifiers cost between $20 and $100, so you can purchase three magnifiers for the price of one pair of standard glasses. You may choose to buy more expensive models or buy more than three, but you can have at least a basic set for about $100 to $200. The exception to this is a video magnifier (CCTV), which is an excellent tool for anyone with less than 20/70 vision. If you have less than 20/400 vision you should definitely consider pur-chasing one. CCTVs use a small projector to mag-nify any type of print or photograph onto a television or monitor screen. Basic single unit models begin at about $1,800. There are several small hand-held models ranging from $400 to $900 that plug into your television. Check with the catalog companies listed in the back of this book, and your local low vision program or retailer for the latest information on video magnifiers (CCTVs).

GOOD ADVICE

Talk to your doctor before you purchase any optical aid that costs more than $500, unless you are purchasing a video magnifier (CCTV). Magnifiers, high-power lenses, special glasses, and telescopes should not be more expensive than a designer pair of regular glasses. They are often less. Ask your doctor about low vision rehabilitation programs in your area where you can get help with these choices, or call the organizations listed in Appendix I for help finding a program.

Choosing the Right Magnifiers

There are two broad categories of magnifiers: magnifiers for seeing up close, and telescopes for seeing things at a distance. To get the right one you need to know what you want it to do, and what the magnifier you are considering actually does. This may sound like common sense, but if you are considering several catalog pages of magnifiers that look alike, it tends to get a bit complicated. This is probably why some catalogs offer a limited selection. If you are ordering on your own, ask your catalog sales representative any questions you may have. Pay particular attention to how close you will have to hold your magnifier, how large an area you will be able to see, and whether or not it will leave both your hands free.

Testing and Returning Magnifiers

Do not buy a magnifier without a return guarantee. You don't want to be stuck with one that doesn't work for you. Reputable catalogs, programs, and dealers will offer you a wide choice, and a free trial period or a full refund within 30 days (except for computer software, which is usually not returnable because it is so easily copied). At Low Vision Living, we loan magnifiers we feel are right for testing at home, often providing several models so that people can choose the particular style that works best for them. Many sales representatives for CCTVs will deliver the equipment to you for testing at no cost. Remember to test your magnifiers as soon as you receive them. Return unwanted ones in their original packaging so they can be resold.

CHOOSING THE RIGHT STRENGTH MAGNIFIER FOR YOU

The first thing to know about buying magnifiers, especially those for seeing up close, is that you shouldn't buy one without knowing what strength you need. The strength of a magnifier is like a prescription in regular glasses, although prescriptions are much more specific. Nevertheless, just as you need to get glasses with the right prescription for them to be useful, you need to get magnifiers in the right strength for them to be useful. The strength of high power reading glasses and magnifiers is measured in diopter powers and X powers.

What Are Diopter Powers and X Powers?

Most reading glasses, high-powered spectacles, and clip-on lenses or loupes are advertised in diopter powers. Diopter powers are written as

"+ some number." You may see reading glasses in drugstores and catalogs labeled +1 or +2, meaning that they are +1 or +2 diopters in strength. Most magnifiers are advertised in X powers, which are written as "some number X." You will see magnifiers labeled 3X, 4X, and so forth. Diopter powers are the official scientific measurement for all lenses. In other words, all lenses have a certain diopter power. Diopter powers are therefore the most reliable and consistent measurement of strength across brands. But not all brands will advertise them. Many simply give X powers, which are calculated from diopters in an effort to give us some practical information. X powers tell us roughly how many times larger a magnifier will make print or an object. So a 3X magnifier will magnify 3 times the original size, if you hold the magnifier near your eye and at the correct distance from the object. X power measurements vary slightly across brands because they are calculated on either an American or a European scale, depending on the manufacturer.

What Diopter Power or X Power Do You Need?

To find the power you need, turn to the Magnifier Selection Chart below and follow these steps:

Finding Your Power with <u>Macular Degeneration</u>'s Magnifier Selection Chart

1. Wear your usual reading glasses and sit in a well-lit area.
2. Hold the Selection Chart 16 inches (40 cm) away.
3. Choose the smallest line you can read comfortably, without straining.
4. Follow the print line across the page to the four columns on the right.

The first two columns tell you what power magnifier you will probably need, measured in both American and European X powers. The third column tells you what power reading glasses you will need, measured in diopters. And the last column gives the visual acuity that usually fits these particular powers.

Determining Your Power by the Print Size You Can Read

<u>MACULAR DEGENERATION</u>'S MAGNIFIER SELECTION CHART

If there is a rehabilitation program in your area, please go. They will help you select magnifiers and train you in their use. If there is no program in your area, this chart is designed for you. Keep in mind that as magnifiers get more powerful, they also get smaller and trickier to use.

Sample Print	Magnifier Powers U.S.	European	Diopters	Visual Acuity
I can do this. It is very hard to do, but if I try my best I will succeed			+2.5	20/30
I can do this. It is very hard to do, but I will try.	1.25X		+4–5	20/50
I can do this. It is very difficult	1.75X	2.5X	+6–7	20/60
I can do this if I try.	2X	3X	+8	20/80
I can do this if I try.	3X	4X	+12	20/100

Remember: magnifiers in powers higher than 6X are quite small. You will need to hold the magnifier and the material very close to your eyes to see a large enough area of print to read. At these high powers, a CCTV is your best option for continuous reading.

SAMPLE PRINT	MAGNIFIER POWERS		DIOPTERS	VISUAL ACUITY
	U.S.	EUROPEAN		
I can do this.	4X	5X	+16	20/125
I can do this.	5X	6X	+20	20/150
I can do this	6X	7X	+24	20/200
I can do it	7X	8X	+28	20/250

I can

9X 10X   +36   20/300

I can

12X 13X   +48   20/400

I will

15X 16X   +60   20/500

When you use the chart, choose your power based on the line you feel most comfortable reading. Do not worry about the visual acuity figures that correspond to this line of print listed on the right of the page. These numbers are there only to provide out-of-town family and friends with a ballpark guesstimate of your magnifier strength. For example, if your friends or family know that your vision is 20/80, they can order a magnifier in the corresponding X power.

When Powers Vary

Magnifier preferences vary among people. Two people who have exactly the same visual acuity measurements may prefer different strength magnifiers. Why? Because the ease with which you read depends not only on your visual acuity but also upon contrast sensitivity. If you have good contrast sensitivity (you can easily distinguish between objects of similar color or of similar lightness or darkness) you will not need as much magnification to read the same line of print as you would if you had less contrast sensitivity. Additionally, practiced readers who have completed *Macular Degeneration*'s Reading Workshop or another visual rehabilitation reading program will not need as much magnification as those who do not read regularly and have had no reading training.

Magnifier preferences may also vary for a

single individual. For example, Dolores Lopez determined from *Macular Degeneration*'s Magnifier Selection Chart that 4X is her correct power. However, she bought a 4X lighted hand-held magnifier and a 5X unlighted hand-held model. Why? Without adequate light Dolores needs a more powerful magnifier. She carries the 5X unlighted model during the day to stores and restaurants that have variable lighting and finds that the 5X gives her enough additional magnification to compensate for less light.

Finally, magnifier powers vary slightly between catalogs because some catalogs list American X powers and some list European X powers. Both American and European powers are listed on the Magnifier Selection Chart. *Macular Degeneration*'s Magnifier Selection Chart provides you with a guideline for choosing the best magnifiers for you, but you may find that you need a power higher or lower than you anticipated. Ordering magnifiers from a catalog is just like ordering clothes from a catalog—it's not an exact science. If you have any questions, double check your order with your optometrist, ophthalmologist or catalog sales representative.

Finding Diopters and Powers for Someone Else

If you are choosing a magnifier for a friend or family member who lives elsewhere or as a surprise gift, you will need to know the correct power or diopter magnifier to buy. If you don't have this information, you can use your friend or family member's 20/20 visual acuity measurement and the Magnifier Selection Chart to estimate the correct power or diopter. If your friend or family member has been told by his or her eye doctor that their vision is "count fingers," this means it is less than 20/400. With 20/400 vision, you will need to buy at least a 12X or a +48 diopter magnifier, or better yet contribute to a video magnifier (CCTV). Always keep your receipt and the original packaging in case the magnifier needs to be returned or exchanged. If you have absolutely no information on your friend or family member's vision, buy another sort of product such as a large button high-contrast telephone, talking calculator, or large print address book. If your heart is set on a magnifier, try buying lightweight binoculars or opera glasses for distance viewing instead of a magnifier for close viewing.

THE MOST COMMON MAGNIFIER MISTAKES

Mistake 1. Any Magnifier Will Work

It is very difficult for fully sighted people to understand that all magnifiers are not created equally. If you have full sight, it *is* true that any magnifier will work for you. Everything will look clear, it will just look bigger or smaller depending on the strength of the magnifier. But if you have macular degeneration, a magnifier that is not strong enough for you will not make everything look clear. Everything will still appear blurry. It won't work. That's why it's so important to buy magnifiers for close viewing in the right diopter or power.

Mistake 2. Bigger Magnifiers Make Things Bigger

The laws of physics dictate that the more powerful the magnifier, the smaller its lens. So bigger magnifiers are also weaker magnifiers. They cover a bigger area, but they don't make things that much bigger. If you find a huge hand-held magnifier in a store or catalog, or a magnifier that enlarges a whole page, you can bet that it's probably a 2X, which means that it will only make print appear two times its original size. If you need more magnification, you will need a smaller magnifier. With a smaller magnifier, you will see better, but you will see less print at a time.

Mistake 3. Stronger Magnifiers Are Better

Do not buy the strongest magnifier on the market. Instead, buy the weakest magnifier you can use without straining. Why? Because the stronger the magnifier is, the smaller its lens, and the less area you will be able to see with it. For example, with a 2X magnifier, you will be able to see the entire line below. With a 5X magnifier, you will see only the first four words. And holding a 7X magnifier, you will only see the first two words before you would have to move the magnifier or the page. It's obviously much easier to read if you can see more words at a time, so you need to opt for the weakest magnifiers you can use without straining.

I can do this, especially if it's sunny. (2X)

I can do this (5X)
I can (7X)

If you are using stronger magnifiers, you can see a few more words at a time if you hold the magnifier very, very close. But you will still not be able to see as many words at a time as you could with a weaker magnifier.

Mistake 4. You Can Hold All Magnifiers at the Same Distance

The stronger the magnifier, the closer you will have to hold it to your eyes and to your reading material. The weaker the magnifier, the farther you can hold it, and the more comfortable reading distance you will have. This is why video magnifiers (CCTVs) are popular. With high-powered loupes (lenses) and glasses, print is in focus only if it's held as close as 1 to 8 inches away from your eyes, depending upon the precise power of the lens. With a video magnifier (CCTV), you can get the same magnification while sitting at a comfortable distance from the screen. Before you order a magnifier or lens in high powers, ask your sales representative how close you will have to hold it, and how close you will have to hold the material you are reading, so you will not be surprised when the product arrives. For high powered reading glasses, your best bet is to have them professionally fitted by an optometrist or ophthalmologist who specializes in low vision.

Mistake 5. Lighting Doesn't Matter

You need good light to see with a magnifier. Magnifiers have solid frames or edges that block light, and your hand, head, or shoulders can block light or cast shadows, especially when you hold material very close to your eyes. When you are evaluating magnifiers, make sure you have bright light directed onto the page. A regular shade lamp with an incandescent lightbulb is almost never a good enough source of light. The bulb disperses the light into the room instead of onto the page, and the shade makes things even worse by muting much of the light, sending the remainder up to the ceiling and down to the floor. A goose-neck or flexible arm lamp with a floodlight bulb is much better. If glare is a problem, adjust the lamp so light shines from the side onto the page, or consider using a lighted magnifier or magnifier mounted on a lamp. If you plan to use your magnifier in public or poorly lit areas where you do not control the light source, consider using a lighted magnifier or carry a lightweight pocket flashlight or penlight. If you feel your magnifier isn't working, always check your lighting first.

CHOOSING A MAGNIFIER FOR CLOSE VIEWING

There are five types of magnifiers for close viewing. Each type can be found in many different styles and strengths. The best type and style for you depends upon the strength you need, what you need the magnifier to do, and your personal preference. Magnifiers for close viewing are harder to choose than ones for distance, because reading is a more precise task. You can see leaves on a tree when they are slightly out of focus, but it's difficult to read print that is slightly out of focus. The recommendations listed below explain your options in greater detail. They reflect the magnifier choices most people find helpful. I will discuss the magnifiers best suited for spot reading (reading small amounts), continuous reading, working with both hands, and writing.

THE FIVE TYPES OF MAGNIFIERS FOR CLOSE VIEWING

1. **Hand-held magnifiers**

2. **Magnifiers in nonadjustable holders that sit directly on the page**
   These include stand magnifiers, paperweight (Brightfield) magnifiers, and bar magnifiers.

3. **Magnifiers on adjustable supports or goosenecks that sit above a page**
   These include lamp magnifiers and the Big Eye.

4. **Electronic magnifiers**
   These include video magnifiers, also called closed-circuit televisions (CCTVs), computer software and hardware.

5. **Magnifiers that sit on your nose or head**
   These include high power glasses, clip-on lenses or loupes, and head-mounted magnifiers, like the Optivisor and Magni-focuser.

Note: Some lenses are called "loupes," which simply means "a lens that magnifies."

Recommendations for Spot Reading (Reading Labels, Addresses, or Small Amounts of Information)

- **Hand-held magnifiers**

For reading labels, price tags, restaurant menus, addresses, meters, dials, and pill bottles, hand-held magnifiers are usually the most convenient option. They come in many sizes, weights, and styles. Lighted ones are very handy for poorly lit public areas; you can purchase electric or battery operated models. Hand-held magnifiers are not as practical for extended reading because they require maintaining a precise, consistent distance from the page. Over time, this may result in arm or wrist fatigue. Hand-held magnifiers are also not practical for doing tasks that require using both hands.

Using a hand-held magnifier

To focus a hand-held magnifier properly, place the magnifier right on the page or object you wish to see. You'll notice that it hardly magnifies when it sits directly on anything. Slowly move the magnifier up from the page until the print comes into focus. If you are using a high power magnifier, which will be small, hold the magnifier close to your eye and to your reading material to see a larger area. A stronger (higher power) magnifier works like a small hole in a fence. If you stand away from the fence you can hardly see anything in the yard beyond. But if you put your eye right up to the hole, you can see almost the entire yard. So, too, with magnifiers.

- **Video magnifiers or closed-circuit televisions (CCTVs)**

  If your vision is less than 20/400, a video magnifier (CCTV) will be the best option for spot reading labels, addresses, notes, and pill bottles and for continuous reading in your home. You can also use it to view photographs. Video magnifiers are also very popular with people who have better vision but would prefer to have a large screen view and a more comfortable reading distance. Video magnifiers use a small projector to enlarge print or an image on a TV screen or monitor. You can vary the level of magnification and the color contrast depending on the size of the monitor you buy and the projector's controls. Some video magnifiers are single units, while others come as a separate camera that you plug into your own TV.

Recommendations for Continuous Reading (Reading Continuously for Longer Periods of Time)

- **Stand magnifiers**

  Stand magnifiers are set in nonadjustable holders that sit directly on a page; they often look like paperweights. You use one of your hands to slide the magnifier across the page. The nice thing about stand magnifiers is that they do not require a steady hand and are not tiring to use. By sitting directly on the page, they automatically maintain a consistent distance from the reading material, so you only have to adjust your eyes. Many stand magnifiers have handles. You can purchase different strength lenses to slide onto the handle. They also come in lighted and unlighted styles. Most stand magnifiers come in up to 8X power, but you can buy a Coil high power stand magnifier in up to 20X or loupe stand magnifiers up to 22X.

If you have fairly good vision, you might like a paperweight (Brightfield) magnifier, which looks like a dome-shaped or slice-shaped glass paperweight. Their design allows them to pull more light onto the page. Bar magnifiers are also popular. They can cover an entire line or page, but they are not very strong and do not attract light.

Using stand magnifiers

Stand magnifiers are easy to focus and do not require a steady hand since they sit right on your reading material. Simply place them on a page and adjust your reading distance. If you are using a higher power magnifier, remember that if you move your eye closer to the page, you will see more print at a time. However, the closer you hold your magnifier, the more important good lighting will be. You may also need to use a reading stand for comfortable posture. You may see better with many stand magnifiers if you also wear your bifocals.

- **Video magnifiers or closed-circuit televisions (CCTVs)**

  If you have less than 20/400 vision, your best option for continuous reading is a video magnifier—also called a CCTV—(see CCTVs under Spot Reading above). Many people with better vision also prefer CCTVs.

- **High-power reading glasses and clip-on lenses (loupes)**

  High-power reading glasses are very complicated to choose correctly, much more complicated than magnifiers. For this reason, many low vision specialists believe they should be prescribed by an optometrist or ophthalmologist like regular glasses, not purchased from catalogs. I am including information about them here for people who do not have access to visual rehabilitation programs or doctors who specialize in low vision.

  High-power reading glasses and lenses are good for sitting and reading or working in a well-lit place with good back and arm support. They are not good for looking around the room or walking. They do allow a larger field of view than equivalent power magnifiers, which means that you can see more words on a page at once, but you must hold material very close to your eyes to read, in some cases as close as one inch. As a result, like loupes, high-power glasses require patience and practice for continuous reading, but many people come to like them.

In addition to high-power glasses, half-eye high-power reading glasses up to +12 diopters are available in low vision catalogs and stores. Full size monocular reading glasses from +14 to +20 diopters are also available. They have one high-power lens and one plain glass lens because they require you to hold material so close that it is too difficult to focus with both eyes; instead, you can use them to read with your best eye. Extremely high power clip-on lenses or loupes are available up to +60 diopters.

Using high-power reading glasses, lenses, and spectacles

To focus properly, start with your reading material right up against your glasses, then move it away until it becomes clear. This is your required reading distance. Make sure that you have good, direct light on the page you are reading, preferably a gooseneck lamp with an indoor floodlight. Regular shade lamps with incandescent bulbs are often not a good enough source of light.

Recommendations for Working with Both of Your Hands

• Optivisor and Magni-focuser

These magnifiers feature lenses in lightweight plastic frames attached to headbands or headsets. The plastic frames flip down over your eyes or regular glasses when you need to see something while using both hands. They are available in up to 4X power. You can also use high-power reading glasses, clip-on lenses, or binocular spectacles for working with both hands, although you would have to take them completely off to walk around.

• The Big Eye

The Big Eye is an adjustable or gooseneck lamp in floor or table models with one or two magnifiers attached. It also comes in a double-neck model with the magnifiers on one and the light on the other. You can position the Big Eye so you are looking through the magnifier with adequate light shining directly on whatever you are viewing.

Recommendations for Writing

• Pen and paper

If you use pink ink and yellow paper, you may have difficulty writing no matter what magnifier you use. Color contrast plays a big role in writing. Do not use colored inks, including reds and blues, pencils, or ballpoint pens because they are difficult to see. Always use black ink-tip or felt-tip pens on white paper. To guide your writing, use dark lined paper or a dark guide sheet. You can also use big-print checks, check registers, calendars, and date books.

- **Optivisor, Magni-focuser, and the Big Eye**

  Many people like to use one of these three for writing.

- **High-power glasses**

  Since you don't need to see as clearly to write well as you do to read, try using glasses for writing that are half the strength you usually need for reading in order to gain more working distance. Very high power reading glasses are not practical for writing because they require you to hold the material too close.

MAGNIFYING COMPUTER SOFTWARE

There are many different options for adapting your computer for low vision. The easiest adjustment to make is to move closer to your monitor. You may need a monitor stand that accommodates a near distance without requiring uncomfortable posture. A moveable monitor arm is also highly recommended. If you move closer to your monitor, you may also need stronger reading glasses. The second easiest adjustment to make is to buy a larger monitor. Moving from a fourteen-inch screen to a twenty-inch screen increases the size of the text by 40 percent, while still allowing you to see the same number of words on the screen at a time.

There are software programs available that will enlarge the text on your screen up to 16X. There are also many talking computer software programs. Because software is so easy to copy, it is usually not returnable, so you will want to be sure you have the right product before you purchase it. Ask whether the system will do exactly what you need, whether the software is compatible with your computer, and whether you have enough space on your hard drive and enough memory (RAM) to store and run the program. Consider checking with your state's commission for the blind or department of rehabilitation for advice and opportunities for computer demonstration and training. See the back of this book for a selected list of computer products and retailers.

TELESCOPES FOR SEEING AT A DISTANCE

Telescopes for seeing at a distance can be extremely useful. Many people use them for reading street signs or airline gate numbers, for examining display cabinets, or for seeing museum pieces. They are much easier to choose than magnifiers for reading, mostly because you don't need to get precisely the correct power magnifier to see well. Most people use either a regular pair of binoculars or a 4X or 8X monocular telescope, regardless of how low their vision may be. There is, however, one additional consideration when choosing distance magnifiers: field of view.

Field of View

As you may know from looking through binoculars, any distance magnifier will have a telescope effect: it will limit the width or field of your view, giving you the impression that you are looking at the world through a tunnel. In general, less than ten degrees of field is not useful. Catalogs will often list the field of view, but if they don't you should ask.

Lens Advertising and Measurements

Monocular telescopes, binoculars, and binocular spectacles are often advertised differently from near-distance lenses. Instead of being advertised as 4X, 8X, or 10X, they will appear as 4X10, 4X12, 8X12, and so forth. The first number indicates the X power of the lens: a 4X, 8X, or 10X lens. The second number indicates the diameter of the outer (objective) lens of the telescope or monocular. The first number divided into the second tells you the physical area in millimeters that you look *through* when you use the lens (not the breadth or field of view that you *see* when you use lens). The larger that area is, the easier the lens will be to focus. For example, a 4X12 lens = 12 divided by 4 = 3 millimeters. This will be easier to focus than a 8X16 lens, which will only give you 2 millimeters.

Recommendations for Reading Street Signs, Building Signs, and Airline Gate Numbers

- **Regular lightweight binoculars, field glasses, or opera glasses**

Since most people have a pair of binoculars or opera glasses, or can purchase an inexpensive pair at a local hardware or camping store, I recommend experimenting with them first. Take them when you leave home. Try spot-reading street signs and watching longer events to get a feel for what you can see, and whether you are comfortable holding them for longer periods of time. If you have trouble seeing, consider stronger monocular telescopes or binocular spectacles. Keep in mind, though, that the stronger the telescope, the heavier it will be and the steadier you will have to hold it.

- **Monocular telescopes, monoculars, and clip-on monoculars**

Monoculars are lenses set in a thick round barrel that you hold up to your eye. They look like telephoto lenses for a camera. You can also purchase tiny ones to clip onto your glasses. If your vision is pretty good, you can use regular binoculars instead. Otherwise, I usually recommend

4X12 with variable focus, which will give you a relatively strong power, a wide field, and a range of distances. In any case, lenses with less than ten degrees of field are usually not useful.

Recommendations for Watching Stage Performances, Sports Events, Lectures, and Television Shows

- **Binocular far distance spectacles**

Binocular spectacles are sometimes called TV glasses or sports glasses in catalogs. The advantage to using them over regular binoculars or telescopes is that you don't have to hold them, so you won't experience arm fatigue. Nevertheless, many people do use regular binoculars or monoculars for extended distance viewing.

A NOTE ON DRIVING

A few states allow people with specific levels of low vision to drive with special, individually fitted bioptic telescopes. These telescopes are mounted on glasses in a position slightly above center, allowing you to read traffic signals and signs. A driver training program is usually required. Check with your secretary of state for your state's regulations. Not all visual rehabilitation programs fit bioptic telescopes for driving. You may have to contact the national organizations listed at the back of this book for the program, optometrist, or ophthalmologist nearest you who fits these lenses.

MAGNIFIER PROBLEMS: MY BACK AND NECK FEEL STRAINED WHEN I READ

Use a Reading Stand or an Adjustable Height Table

For stand magnifiers, reading stands or adjustable tables are almost a necessity. Ideally, you need to position the material and magnifier so it is high enough that your back can remain straight while you read. You may have to create an individual reading station for comfortable continuous reading. You can combine a reading stand with an adjustable height table, or use the table for a CCTV. Some low vision catalogs carry stands and tables, or you can purchase them at an office supply store or a medical supply store. Hospital-type bed tables actually work very well as CCTV stands.

WHY WON'T MY MAGNIFIER WORK?

Possibility 1. Not Enough Light

Regular shade lamps and regular indoor lighting are often not good enough. I recommend a gooseneck lamp, either a table or floor model, with an indoor floodlight bulb. Goosenecks are adjustable, allowing you to direct light onto the page, and floodlight bulbs provide much more concentrated light than regular incandescent bulbs. Alternatively, consider a lighted magnifier or the Big Eye.

Possibility 2. The Wrong Strength Magnifier

If you have a magnifier that is too weak, it won't be useful. Double-check your correct power with *Macular Degeneration*'s Magnifier Selection Chart and compare your correct power to the magnifier's power. If you purchased the magnifier at a drugstore and do not know its power, it is safe to assume that it is not more than 3X, and probably less.

Possibility 3. Your Scotoma Is Getting in the Way (see Chapter 10 for Scotomas)

If you are trying to use damaged areas of your central vision (your scotoma) to see, rather than maximizing your best areas of vision, your magnifier will not work as well. See Chapter 10, Your Reading Workshop, for a complete guide to finding your scotoma and learning to move it out of the way through reading practice. In general, reading practice will help you use your magnifiers more effectively to see anything, not just to read. If you haven't done the workshop, give it a try!

CHAPTER 13

Saving Sight in Your Home

I have a simple philosophy. Fill what's empty. Empty what's full. And scratch where it itches.
    —Alice Roosevelt Longworth

Who shall say I am not the happy genius of my household?
    —William Carlos Williams

Your home is your haven. There at least, you can arrange your shelves the way you like them, put floodlights in the living room, and turn up the radio. This chapter will help you arrange your home for maximum visibility and ease. It begins with a few tips that will be helpful for the whole house, and then looks at each room and makes more specific suggestions. For more detailed lighting and magnifier advice, please see Chapters 11 and 12.

FOR EVERY ROOM IN YOUR HOME

Increasing Contrast and Decreasing Pattern

If you have macular degeneration, increasing contrast will make any object immediately more visible. Increasing contrast means increasing the color or dark-light contrast between an object and its background. For example, a black pen on a white tablecloth has great contrast, while a black pen on a black tablecloth has no contrast. Objects that do not contrast with their backgrounds may disappear. A white salt shaker on a white table cloth might as well be wearing camouflage in the jungle. The idea is to increase contrast wherever you can in your home. There are many ways to do so. For example, if certain doorways, furniture, or stairs are difficult to see, have them painted contrasting colors and use contrasting chair covers or tablecloths. For hard-to-see glass coffee tables, put a brightly colored coffee table book on the edge of the table to make it more visible.

Decreasing pattern means decreasing color confusion (which is essentially another way to increase contrast). Pattern means multicolored fabrics or backgrounds. Flowered plates, tablecloths, bedsheets, and bank checks are examples of pattern. Patterns provide terrible contrast.

Peas on a pretty flowered plate will be much harder to find than peas on a white plate. Similarly, a utensil or pen will be harder to find on a plaid tablecloth than on a plain contrasting one. While you're increasing contrast in your home, try to decrease pattern, too.

Labeling and Organizing

Now you can use the labeling supplies you collected for this chapter (see Chapter 9). Just about anything in your home can be labeled, including meters, switches, clothing, clothing hangers, bottles, and boxed or canned goods. You don't have to label everything, though. Often you can use organizing instead of labeling to help you identify items quickly. For example, if you put chicken soup cans in one row, split pea in a second row, and minestrone in a third, you don't have to label the cans to know which is which. You can also distinguish brown socks from blue socks by keeping them in separate drawers and washing them in separate netted hosiery bags. Labeling, however, can be especially valuable for hard-to-see dials and buttons or for things you absolutely don't want to mix up, like prescription medications. When labeling, try to simplify by marking only the most frequently used dial settings or buttons (300 and 350 degrees on your stove, for example, or the preferred room temperature on your thermostat).

Open Space

Don't save things. I know it's tempting, but it will cause you more headaches than it will spare. Extra jars, stockpiled canned goods, old files, and unused clothing all create clutter and crowd closets and shelves. Blocked pathways and objects piled on steps are hazardous. Clearing as much open space as possible in your home will make everything easier to locate, it will make your home easier to clean, and it may be safer. If you are concerned about waste, recycle your containers and contribute your clothing to charity, but don't save.

Predictability

Predictability in your home is enormously important if you have macular degeneration. You can compensate for a lot of sight with predictability. The more predictable your home is, the better. You will always know where everything is. For small items that move around a lot, like house keys, wallets, and glasses, designate a spot for them and try to return them to that spot whenever you come home or put them aside. If you always do, you'll never have to spend an hour searching.

Finding Things

If you drop a pen on the floor or find yourself looking for a bottle of catsup that could be anywhere in the refrigerator, scan systematically. To find the pen, sweep your hands along the floor from right to left, or from your knees outward. To find the catsup, begin searching at the top or bottom of the refrigerator and work your way from left to right on each shelf. If the catsup bottle continues to disappear (which can happen if you are living with someone else), try labeling it with a rubber band so you will know it when you touch it, and assign it an agreed-upon location in the refrigerator.

Lighting and Magnifiers

Good glare-free lighting is essential for seeing just about anything in your home, and magnifiers are often helpful. See Chapter 11 for advice on improving lighting, and Chapter 12 for advice on magnifiers. For detailed work or reading small print in any room you may find a small gooseneck lamp with an indoor floodlight bulb and a small, lightweight flashlight helpful. You may also find a wide range of hand-held and stand magnifiers, lighted magnifiers, and magnifying lamps very helpful.

SELECTED HELPFUL PRODUCTS

Lists of selected helpful products are highlighted in boxes throughout the chapter. These lists are not comprehensive. They are meant to suggest the wide range of products available through the low vision catalogs listed at the end of the book. If you are hearing impaired, you may need talking books and products with male voices, since female voices with higher pitches may be difficult to hear.

LIVING ROOM AND FAMILY ROOM

Living rooms and family rooms are often dimly lit or bathed in bright sunlight. Either extreme may make it very difficult for you to see well enough to enjoy watching television or using a magnifier to read. Adapt the light in these rooms with good lamps, and sheer curtains or blinds. Reduce glare by covering shiny surfaces with tablecloths or heavy, secured area rugs, or by wearing yellow- or plum-tinted glasses (see Chapter 11).

SELECTED HELPFUL PRODUCTS

Television screen enlarger
Large-button remote control

Large-print books, crossword puzzles,
Audiobooks, *Newsweek,* and *Reader's
Digest* on tape
National Public Radio, sports radio
broadcasts

Automatic needle threader, self-
threading needles
Big print measuring tape

Televisions

- Position your television away from reflecting
or bright light, and *sit close to it.* If you still
have trouble seeing the screen, try Coil
focusable telescope glasses or a screen
enlarger. Screen enlargers sit directly in
front of your television, magnifying the
whole screen by about 25 percent, although
they also give you a narrow viewing angle.
Use a large button remote control for newer
television sets. If you have an old set, mark
your favorite stations on your television dial

with a permanent marker or high contrast puff paint.

- Watch national or public television news broadcasts (which have both national and local news programs), but avoid local network news, especially if you live in large cities or metropolitan areas. Local network news tends to sensationalize crime and foster fear. It's stressful to watch and it doesn't provide you with an accurate picture of the community. If you want to hear the sports and weather reports, turn the news on halfway through the broadcast or listen to radio sports and weather broadcasts.

Armchair or Couch Reading

If you want to sit on a favorite chair or couch and use a magnifier to read, you may need to make a few adjustments.

- With high-power reading glasses, prop your elbows on the arms of the chair to comfortably maintain a closer reading distance.

- Make sure adequate light is shining directly on the page. Most people prefer a strong floor lamp or gooseneck table lamp with an indoor floodlight.

- A stand magnifier requires a solid base, so you will need to use a clipboard, lap desk, or ideally a variable-height pull-up table on casters that can hold a reading stand. A pull-up table with good light can also be used for writing or crossword puzzles. Alternatively, you may find it easier to read at a table you already own. If so, consider purchasing a comfortable desk chair to match.

The Library of Congress Talking Books Program

- The National Library Service (NLS) lends books on tape at no charge to people with low vision. Postage for returning the tapes is also free. The NLS offers a wonderfully wide selection of books. New titles are announced in semimonthly catalogs. NLS books on tape must be played on a four-track tape player, which comes free of charge with your tapes. To join the NLS program, see the information listed at the back of this book.

The *Newsweek* and *Reader's Digest* on Tape Program

- The American Printing House for the Blind offers *Newsweek* and *Reader's Digest* on four-track cassette tapes at no charge for people with low vision. You can play these tapes on an NLS tape player or on your own four-track cassette tape player. You do not have to return the tapes. To join the APHB's program, see the information listed at the back of this book.

Talking Books at Your Bookstore or Local Library

- There are literally thousands of books available on tape through your local bookstore. If you want to read it, it's probably on tape. Every bestseller you can think of, and hundreds of classics, histories, autobiographies, biographies, mysteries, westerns, romances, self-help, and religious or inspirational books can be purchased on tape, although they tend to run between $12 and $25. On-line bookstores are another good source. Many local libraries also have extensive audiobook collections. For store-bought or local library tapes, you can use a standard inexpensive tape player. If you would like to slow the pace of the tape so the speaker's voice is easier to understand, you can purchase a hand-held or table-top cassette player with a variable speed feature.

Tape Players, Radios, and Stereos

- Many people find those little black buttons on most electronics very difficult to see. Mark the on-off and play buttons with colored tape or sticky labels. You can also label your CDs with a thick permanent marker or put large-print sticky letters on the cases.

- Radio is an excellent source of sports broadcasts, news, interview programs, religious programs, and concerts. Try the National Public Radio station in your area for a wide variety of programming.

Pianos and Musical Instruments

- You do not have to give up music because of low vision, especially instruments you have played for many years. Enlarge sheet music on a copy machine or order big print copies. Increase the amount of light shining directly on your sheet music by using a gooseneck clip or stand lamp with an indoor floodlight.

Armchair or Couch Crafts

- To secure additional light and magnification while having both hands free, consider using a gooseneck floor lamp with a mounted magnifier that can be placed next to your work and adjusted as necessary. Check the magnification available on these lamps with your own magnifying needs when ordering. You can also use them in combination with reading glasses.

- Use color contrast to make needlework or other crafts more visible to you. Knit or crochet light yarn with dark needles, and dark yarn with white needles. Sew dark buttons on with white thread and use a permanent marker to darken the thread afterward. If you are using light yarn or thread, put a solid dark towel or cloth in your lap. If you are using dark yarn or thread, put a solid white towel or cloth in your lap. Avoid working with pastels or colors that you have difficulty seeing.

- Use a needle threader or stick a self-threading needle into a bar of soap for stability while you thread it.

KITCHEN AND DINING ROOM

Kitchens can easily become cluttered. Before you start cooking, clear away as much as you can, discard unused jars, and avoid overstuffing your shelves. It's more important to be able to see what you have, than to have a lot that you can't see. Make sure you have clearly lit counter space. Use towels or placemats to cut countertop glare and consider replacing irritating overhead fluorescent lights with indoor floodlights. Fluorescent fixtures mounted under kitchen cabinets can be effective since the bulb is not exposed and so produces less glare.

SELECTED HELPFUL PRODUCTS

Large-print cookbooks
Large-print measuring cup
Color coded measuring spoons
Beeping liquid level indicator
Milk carton holder with handle
Large-print timer
Black and white cutting boards
Solid black or navy blue place setting
Solid white place setting

Recipes and Cookbooks

- Use a large-print cookbook, like the large-print version of *In the Kitchen with Rosie* by Rosie Daley, Oprah Winfrey's chef. You can order large-print cookbooks through low vision catalogs or bookstores. You can also make your own large-print cookbook by reprinting your recipes with a thick black marker on 8.5-by-11-inch paper and collecting them in a three-ring binder. Alternatively, enlarge your recipes on a photocopier or print them in large letters with a computer. Enlarge the recipes in Chapter 4 with a photocopier and add them to your collection.

Cooking

- Use color contrast, your sense of smell and touch, and big-print or talking timers or clocks to help you cook. If you have trouble seeing certain foods, use either a light or dark cutting board for background contrast. Prepare onions on a dark board, for example, and red peppers on a white one.

- Consider grouping the items that you are cooking with on a plastic tray to keep them handy and organized. And use a portable gooseneck lamp for additional light.

Pouring and Measuring

- To avoid or minimize spills, set your glass or bowl in the sink when you pour. When you are pouring from a container, rest the lip of the container on the edge of the glass for more stability, especially for hot liquids. Don't fill glasses or cups to the top. With cold liquids, slip your finger over the edge of the glass and stop pouring when you feel the liquid at your finger. With hot liquids, consider using a beeping liquid level indicator. Use coffee mugs with lids. Drink coffee from a white mug, and milk from a dark one.

- Use a big-print measuring cup or mark the cup and half cup lines on your glass measuring cup with a black permanent marker. Or use graduated colored measuring cups or spoons to distinguish between different amounts or mark your measuring equipment with different colored stickers.

Using Ovens and Appliances

- Mark your appliance buttons or dials with a black permanent pen, black or white tape, or sticky labels. It may be easiest to mark only the settings that you use most frequently. For example, 300 and 350 on your oven, high, medium, and low on your burners, and selected buttons on your microwave.

- If you purchase new appliances, check the buttons and dials for visibility. They should be large and have large print or good color contrast. Sometimes fancy digital appliances are much more difficult to see than cheaper models. Choose stoves with easily accessible dials at the front.

- Use oven mitts instead of hand-held hotpads to reduce your risk of accidental burns. Always pull the oven rack out before you place or remove pans. Listen for a click or double-check your appliances when you turn them off.

Dining at Home

- Consider using either dark or light solid color plates and leave flowered plates on a shelf. Purchase a place setting of inexpensive white plastic dishes, and a place setting of navy blue or black ones. Eat light colored foods on the dark plates and dark colored foods on the light plates. For example, serve mashed potatoes in a navy blue bowl and serve spinach salad on a white plate. Drink coffee from a white mug and milk from a dark mug.

- Consider using a solid-color table cloth that contrasts with your plates. Avoid flowered or plaid table cloths since plates, condiments, and pens are more difficult to see against patterned backgrounds. Cream, black, navy blue, and bright gold or orange are generally the best tablecloth colors.

- Put foods that roll easily, like peas or corn, in bowls (as you would with fresh blueberries).

BEDROOMS AND BATHROOMS

Contrast can be particularly helpful in the bedroom and bathroom for distinguishing between items. Good lighting is, of course, always helpful, especially in bathrooms where glare can be a problem, or in closets where you may need more light.

SELECTED HELPFUL PRODUCTS

Big-print or talking clocks or watches
Magnifying mirror
Colored plastic trays and bins
Contrasting toothbrush and
    toothpaste
Contrasting towels and soap

Clocks and Watches

- Avoid digital clocks and watches with poorly lit displays. Most of them use large red or tiny black numbers against deep gold backgrounds, which are extremely difficult to see. Instead, opt for black and white large-print or talking clocks, alarms, and watches. Put one in each room as needed.

Personal Care

- Label look-alike bottles with permanent markers or large-print sticky letters. Wind a rubber band around a bottle to distinguish it from others. Alternatively, designate places for your bottles on different shelves or in different rooms. For example, keep your deodorant on a middle shelf and your moisturizer on a bottom shelf. You may also want to use brightly colored plastic organizer trays to keep items separate and quickly identifiable.

- Use color contrast to make the bathroom and yourself more visible. If your bathroom is white, use solid dark primary colored towels, toothbrushes, toothpaste, and soap. Use the bathroom mirror for combing your hair and hang a solid colored towel behind your head for contrast. If

you have light hair, hang a dark towel;
if you have dark hair, hang a white
towel.

- For shaving and applying makeup, use your
fingers to feel for unshaven areas or to guide
your hand to your eyes or lips. Remember,
it's always easier to aim for the fingers of
your opposite hand than to aim for anything
else. You may also want to use a magnifying
makeup mirror. For clipping nails, rest your
hands on a contrasting cloth. You may also
want to use a gooseneck lamp with an
attached magnifier.

Clothing

- Use safety pins to distinguish between navy
blue, dark green, and black clothing. Place
one pin in navy clothing, two in dark green,
and none in black. Pin or clip socks together
for the laundry. Keep dark colored clothes
sorted in your closet: navy on one side, black
on the other, and green in the middle, or
separate them by a white shirt. You can also
use black, white, or brightly colored plastic
bins to distinguish sweaters or socks. When
you buy new clothing, consider choosing one
base color, either navy, brown, or black, and
purchasing most of your shoes, socks, pants,
or skirts in this color.

- If you have difficulty matching clothes, try carrying your options into sunlight during the day, where color differences will be more visible. Improve the lighting in your closet or use a hand-held flashlight or lighted low-power hand magnifier. Use clothing tags to tell whether clothes are right side out and facing forward.

LAUNDRY AND CLEANING

- If your washer and dryer are in a basement or dark closet, or if they have small dials, you will need good lighting. Some people find flashlights or clip-on gooseneck lamps that can be aimed directly at machine dials to be particularly helpful. You may also want to mark the "on," "off," and your most frequently used wash or dry cycle buttons or points on the dial with permanent markers or sticky tape.

- Tell your dry cleaner that you have low vision and ask him or her to label navy blue, black, and pastel clothing for you with safety pins or by grouping hangers together. If your cleaner is unresponsive, try arriving at the least busy times of the day, or choose a cleaner who is friendlier.

- Use a regular pattern for ironing, housecleaning, and yard work. Just as you would mow the lawn in even regular strips so as not to miss a patch of grass, iron, dust, or sweep in regular patterns. When ironing, you can also use a contrasting ironing board cover to make clothing easier to see. Wear an oven mitt to avoid accidental burns. Never iron with poor lighting. Avoid big ironing or cleaning jobs by folding laundry as soon as it dries, and by cleaning once a week regardless of whether you can see dust or dirt.

- Clearly label toxic substances and try to avoid using them. We usually don't need powerful ammonias, bleaches, bug sprays, and plant pesticides to have a clean home and healthy plants.

HEALTHCARE

- Use color contrast to tell pills apart by marking the bottles with puff paint, black or white tape, or brightly colored stickers. Or use rubber bands to tell them apart by touch. Keep medication that you frequently confuse in different rooms or on different shelves.

- Keep a 4-by-6-inch white index card for each prescription medication. Use a black marker to write down the prescription information and as many slash marks as there are refills allotted. As you reorder, cross each slash mark. The remaining slashes will remind you of the number of refills that you have left. Keep all your index cards together with a big ring clip that you can purchase at an office supply store.

SELECTED HELPFUL PRODUCTS

Talking weight scale and thermometer
Talking blood pressure meter
Big-print weekly pill boxes
Big-print insulin syringes and syringe
  magnifiers

OUTLETS, THERMOSTATS, AND THERMOMETERS

- To insert electric plugs into outlets, place one finger on the outlet. Hold the plug in your other hand with the prongs aligned and aim the plug toward your finger. If it doesn't fit, rotate the plug 180 degrees and try again. If you still have difficulty, make sure that you have adequate light and try to get your eyes down to the level of the plug.

SELECTED HELPFUL PRODUCTS

Large-print thermostat dial
Large-print or talking thermometer

- Mark your preferred room temperature on your thermostat with a permanent marker or purchase a boldface thermostat dial. You can also purchase a big-print or talking thermostat, or a magnifier that fits over your thermostat dial.

CALENDARS, CORRESPONDENCE, AND TELEPHONES

- Use large-print telephone and address books. You can also make your own by reprinting your current books on white 8.5-by-11-inch paper with black permanent marker. Organize these sheets in a handy three ring binder, separated by big-print lettered dividers. You can also print your telephone numbers and addresses in large letters with a computer.

SELECTED HELPFUL PRODUCTS

Large-print calendars and datebooks
Large-print telephone and address books
Black ink or felt-tip pens

Large-button or voice-activated telephones
Free directory service and operator assistance

- Always use black felt-tip or ink pens on white paper, and ask your friends and family members to use black felt-tip or ink pens on white paper when they leave messages or write you letters. Do not use ballpoint pens, colored ink pens, or pencils. They are much more difficult to see.

- Use a big-button telephone. Be sure to choose one with good color contrast: either white numbers on a black background or black numbers on a white background. Many catalogs offer big-button phones in white with gray numbers, which are no easier to see than those on regular phones. Mark the automatic speed dial buttons on your phone with bright tape, colored stickers, or a permanent marker. You may also like a voice-activated phone that automatically dials the person whose name you say into the receiver. Keep a white pad of paper and a black permanent marker next to the phone for messages.

- Create a large-print directory for your speed-dial pad or large-print labels for automatic dialing buttons.

CHAPTER 14

Saving Sight
in Your Community

**Give to the world the best you have,
and the best will come back to you.**
                              —Madeline Bridge

**Life is either a daring adventure or
nothing at all.**

                              —Helen Keller

Life is a daring adventure! Leave your self-consciousness in your closet, and take your courage and your confidence with you. Venturing out of the house always entails risk. But no one in the world cares about whether we make mistakes except us. If we can make them freely, with patience and humor, we allow others to relax, too. This chapter was designed to be read along with Chapter 6, which discusses social interactions, taking risks, and building connections to your community.

A WORD ABOUT WHITE CANES AND LOW VISION BUTTONS

White identification canes are like magic. They increase your safety on the street by alerting motorists that you may not see them, and they increase your safety on sidewalks, too. White canes also have a salutary effect on people. They encourage altruistic behavior, and they discourage impatience. And a white cane can be a tremendously effective way to say "I have low vision" without having to explain. Many people are reluctant to use white canes, fearing vulnerability. But according to the American Foundation for the Blind, carrying a white cane does not increase your risk of crime.

You may be thinking, *What? Me with a white cane? You've got to be kidding!* Many of my patients tell me exactly that. We so closely associate white canes with the profoundly blind, with vulnerability, and with looking conspicuous, that carrying one does not usually fit our self-image. But it works. It really does. And many of the very same patients who were ready to fire me as their doctor when I suggested a white cane now swear by it, even if they use it only at dusk, for crossing major intersections, or in airports.

White identification canes are only for signaling others, particularly drivers, not for tapping sidewalks or supporting your weight. They come in foldable models that you can carry in a purse, bag, or briefcase and use when needed. They are shorter than the canes that the blind use and lighter than regular canes used for walking support.

Low Vision Buttons

A low-profile alternative to alert others is an "I have low vision" button. Keep one with you and pin it to your coat or sweater when you shop, dine out, or travel. We give them to our patients and they've been very popular. If you would like an "I have low vision" button, you can order one for $1.50 from the National Association for the Visually Handicapped, listed in Appendix I.

LEAVING HOME

- Make sure your front walk, porch, and foyer are well lit. These areas are often dark, making keyholes and alarms very difficult to see. Remember to turn on your porch light, and perhaps your foyer light, before you leave home if you anticipate returning after dark. You may want to install outdoor floodlights on the porch and indoor floodlights in the foyer. Consider putting your outdoor lights on timers or motion-sensitive switches so that they are always on at night or will automatically turn on when you or someone else comes to your porch.

- Take a pocket magnifier and a small penlight or flashlight with you for reading menus, price tags, and bills. Camping stores may be better sources for these lights than hardware stores, which tend to sell bulkier models.

SELECTED HELPFUL PRODUCTS

Lists of selected helpful products are highlighted in boxes throughout the chapter. These lists are not comprehensive. They are meant to suggest the wide range of products available through the low vision catalogs listed at the end of this book. If you are hearing impaired, you may need talking books and products with male voices, since female voices with higher pitches may be difficult to hear.

SELECTED HELPFUL PRODUCTS

White identification cane
Binoculars or monocular telescope

Lightweight shopping cart with
   wheels
Adult tricycle with basket
Battery-operated scooter

WALKING, RIDING, AND CROSSING STREETS

- Follow the green grass edges down sidewalks. If there is no grass, follow someone else going in the same direction. Remember that walking on uneven terrain or bumpy sidewalks will be easier in bright sunlight than at dawn or dusk. Sometimes shadows from buildings and trees are confusing. Be aware of your surroundings.

- Cross at intersections with traffic lights whenever possible. Look for pedestrian crossing buttons on poles near the intersection. Begin crossing the intersection after traffic going in your direction also begins to cross the intersection. At intersections with complicated traffic light patterns, like those with left-turn-only lanes or five-way intersections, memorize the traffic pattern so you can anticipate when you will be able to cross with the light. Consider carrying a white cane with you, and using it for busy intersections or if you are walking at dusk.

- Use lightweight binoculars or a monocular telescope to read street signs and traffic lights.

- Since walking is such good exercise, try to walk as much as possible. If you like to combine walking with shopping, consider taking a lightweight collapsible metal shopping cart if carrying purchases becomes too cumbersome.

CAUTION

Riding adult tricycles or battery-operated scooters may not be advisable for you. Consult with your doctor first and weigh your risks carefully.

- If you live in an area with safe low-traffic streets and good sidewalks, and you've enjoyed bike riding before, consider riding an adult tricycle for exercise or trips to the store. Ride your tricycle on the sidewalk and cross streets at crosswalks. Although tricycles are very stable, you may want to explore routes with a friend or family member the first time you ride in order to avoid potholes and high curbs. Beware of cars backing out of driveways and small children.

- Battery-operated scooters are an alternative for people who have trouble walking or riding a tricycle. They are also convenient for carrying purchases home. Scooters are designed to be driven on sidewalks at walking speed. They have become so popular that the media have reported scooter traffic jams in some senior communities. Some grocery stores provide scooters for their customers. Again, beware of cars backing out of driveways and small children.

BUSES, TAXIS, AND SUBWAYS

If you have always used public transportation, taking the subway or bus with low vision may be challenging. If you have always driven a car, public transportation may be a new experience altogether. Either way, use the one-two-three

SELECTED HELPFUL PRODUCTS

Taxi-hailing card or bus mitten
Photocopy-enlarged bus or subway
   schedule
Local senior transportation services

method for familiarizing yourself with the routes you will take. The first time you use the bus or subway, go with a friend or family member and let them show you how to do it. The second time, go with a friend or family member, but let them simply tag along; make all the decisions yourself. If you have no difficulties on the second trip, the third time you'll be ready to go on your own.

- If you live in New York City or another city with many taxis and many competitive customers, consider carrying a neon yellow card at least 5-by-8-inches high with the word TAXI written in large black print. Hold the card up when you need a ride, and a taxi will find you. You can make one yourself or order one from a low vision catalog.

- If you live in a metropolitan area with fewer taxis and you have friends with low vision, consider scheduling a regular weekly or biweekly shared taxi ride to lunch, the hair stylist, shopping centers, or religious services. Taxi companies in low traffic areas tend to be more responsive to regular or prescheduled customers than to last-minute calls. They are not always prompt, either. Build in a certain amount of additional time so that you aren't rushed.

- Ask your bus company for a bus mitten. Bus mittens look like oven mitts with the company's or transportation authority's logo. They signal the bus driver even before you see the bus coming. They are particularly good for areas where buses do not automatically stop but must be signaled.

- Call your public transportation authority for bus and subway maps and schedules. If they arrive in small print, enlarge them on a photocopy machine and familiarize yourself with the routes and schedules that will be most helpful to you. Many transportation authorities will give you specific route information and times over the phone if you call and tell them that you are visually impaired and need to use the bus to travel to a particular place.

- Bus drivers are often required to assist riders by announcing stops by name. Many drivers will try to be especially helpful if they know that you have low vision. Carry a white identification cane to bus stops or tell the driver that you cannot see well. Double-check by asking the driver when you board whether the bus goes to the stop you need. Sit at the front so that you can hear the driver clearly, and so that he or she doesn't forget that you are there.

- Some cities offer special transportation services for seniors, as do some churches, mosques, synagogues, senior centers, and neighborhood centers. Check with your clergy or county or city offices for more information. Plan ahead when using these services. They are usually low cost, but they may run late and require patience.

MONEY, CHECKS, AND BANKING

Money

- Use a multicompartment billfold or arrange your bills in your wallet according to their value. Keep $1 bills straight, fold $5 bills in half horizontally so they are long and thin, fold $10 in half vertically so they are square, and fold $20 at the right corner. Avoid carrying $50 or $100 bills whenever possible.

- Memorize the sizes and shapes of coins. The edges of quarters and dimes have ridges, but quarters are of course much larger. Nickels and pennies both have smooth edges. You can tell them apart because nickels are thicker and heavier while pennies are smaller and copper colored.

- When wearing clothing with three pockets, keep pennies in one pocket, quarters in another, and dimes and nickels in a third. My father uses this strategy every day and finds it convenient. Alternatively, use a multicompartment change purse.

SELECTED HELPFUL PRODUCTS

Multicompartment billfolds and
    change purses
Hand-held magnifiers

Black ink and felt-tip pens
Large-print checks and check registers
Large-print bank statements
Talking calculator

Checks and Banking

- You can order large-print checks and check registers from your bank. Large-print checks fit easily into legal sized envelopes and are acceptable to creditors and businesses. Many banks provide these checks free of charge to their low vision clients, and many people rave about them.

- If you prefer regular-size checks, choose a plain design with black type. Avoid checks with flowers, pictures, or pastel colors. Check-writing guides for your regular-size checks are available from low vision catalogs, although most people prefer large-print checks. These guides are black templates with oblong slots cut out of them. They fit over your entire check, covering everything except the lines on which you write.

- If you are writing checks at home, use a lamp magnifier like the Big Eye and high-power reading glasses half the strength you normally need to read. Lower strength glasses will give you a more comfortable writing distance. They still work well for writing since you do not need to see quite as clearly to write as you do to read.

- Use a photocopy machine to englarge your bank statement and a talking calculator to

reconcile your statement or checkbook. You
can also use a video magnifier (CCTV) or
regular magnifiers to read printed
statements, or combine personal banking
computer software with screen enlargement
or talking computer software. Some banks
and utility companies offer large-print
statements as a service to their customers.

SELECTED HELPFUL PRODUCTS

Portable gooseneck lamp with indoor
   floodlight bulb
Hand and stand magnifiers
High-power reading glasses

Large-button or voice-activated
   telephone
Dictaphone
Talking calculator
Large-face watches
Black felt-tip or ink pens
Large-print keyboard labels
Computer monitor magnifier
Screen enlargement software and
   hardware
Talking computer and screen reader
   software
Closed-circuit television (CCTV)

JOBS, VOLUNTEER WORK, AND HOME OFFICES

- Do not assume that vision loss means unemployment or an inability to volunteer or be active in community service. Seniors with low vision work as attorneys, professors, company owners, political activists, counselors, hospital greeters, patient visitors, reading tutors, and much more. Use the advice in Part II and the resources listed in the Appendices to help you approach colleagues and organizations with confidence.

SUPERMARKETS AND NEIGHBORHOOD GROCERIES

- Supermarkets are generally organized in the same fashion nationwide. Produce, dairy products, bread, meat, fish, deli and bakery counters are usually located around the perimeter of the store. Boxed, canned, and paper goods are located in the aisles. Familiarize yourself with the layout of your favorite store, the location of your favorite brands, and their appearance. Many brands have distinctively colored labels that make them easier to identify. Campbell's soup, for example, has a striking red and white label.

- Use your hand-held magnifier to read labels and prices.

- Consider contacting the supermarket manager and requesting prearranged assistance. Many supermarkets offer this service to their customers. Neighborhood groceries and delis may also have delivery service or take telephone orders for pickup. Supermarkets and groceries are often short staffed during rush times, usually evenings and weekends, so try to shop weekdays. You are likely to get much better service with less hassle.

- Make a large-print shopping list with a black felt-tip pen and dark lined paper. Arrange the items on the list according to the organization of the store. Alternatively, create a large-print computer generated check-off grocery list that you can photocopy and use every week (or ask a relative or friend to create one).

CLOTHING AND PRODUCT SHOPPING

- Call stores ahead of time to see if they have a particular item in stock or to prearrange sales assistance. Shop at off-peak hours whenever possible. Sales staff often appreciate your effort to come when they aren't rushed.

- Take your pocket flashlight, penlight, hand-held magnifier, or lighted magnifier to see prices, clothing colors, product information, and receipts.

- If you have any questions, don't hesitate to ask. Always inquire about return policies before purchasing products. Some stores have store-credit-only or no-return policies advertised on small placards that you may not see.

RESTAURANTS

- You are most likely to get the best service at off-peak hours: generally before 12:00 or after 1:30 for lunch, and before 6:00 or after 8:30 for dinner. Since off-peak hours vary depending on the restaurant and the area, call ahead of time and ask the staff, or familiarize yourself with customer rush patterns at your favorite restaurants.

- Choose well-lit restaurants and reserve or request tables in well-lit spaces or near sunny windows. Sit with your back or side to the window or light source to maximize light on your menu and plate and to minimize

glare in your eyes. Wear light yellow glasses
to reduce glare. If the light at your table is
uncomfortable or inadequate, explain the
problem to the wait staff and request
reseating. If you are extremely glare-
sensitive, you may actually prefer dining in
darker areas or away from windows.

- To read menus, take your penlight or small
  flashlight, a pocket or purse-size magnifier,
  or lighted hand-held magnifier with you.
  Many menus use very small print and are
  difficult to read, but they may have larger
  print headings for general categories, like
  sandwiches, soups, pastas, vegetarian,
  chicken entrees, and specials. Narrow your
  choice down to a particular category and
  work your way through the list with your
  magnifier. Alternatively, ask your waiter to
  tell you your options in that category or to
  recommend a dish. You can borrow menus
  from your favorite restaurants, enlarge them
  at a photocopy shop, and carry them with
  you or read them at home on your CCTV
  before you dine out.

- Wearing an "I have low vision" button may
  help your waiter recognize that you may not
  see everything. Remember that they are
  there to serve you. You can ask your waiter
  to serve difficult-to-control foods like peas in

separate bowls or to cut meats before they are served to you. When your dish arrives, feel free to ask your waiter or your friend to tell you exactly what is on the plate and where it is.

PARTIES AND CARDS

SELECTED HELPFUL PRODUCTS

Large-print playing cards

Large-print Uno, Rook, and Bingo cards

Large-print Scrabble and Monopoly

Uniquely shaped, high contrast poker chips

Uniquely shaped, high contrast chess and checker sets

- Remember that people come to parties to meet you and enjoy your company. They are usually much more concerned about feeling comfortable themselves or appearing attractive than about whether or not you have low vision. And you have much more to offer a party than how much you can or can't see.

Introduce yourself freely and tell people that you will not be able to recognize their faces so they must introduce themselves in return.

- Your host will want you to enjoy yourself, too, but may have a difficult time anticipating your needs. Put yourself and your host at ease by asking questions and communicating directly. Feel free to ask for a plate with a rim or a bowl for hors d'oeuvres. Do not hesitate to ask for guided directions to the bar or bathroom.

- Ask your friends to play poker, bridge, or other games with big-print cards. These cards are the same size as a regular deck and everyone will find them easier to see.

- Bring a portable gooseneck lamp with a floodlight bulb for the playing table. Everyone will appreciate the additional light. You can also take the same lamp to private clubs. Friends want your company, and private clubs are for members. Living with low vision means letting the world know what you need, and helping people meet those needs. When you feel comfortable, everyone around you will feel more comfortable, too.

GOLF, BOWLING, AND EXERCISE

SELECTED HELPFUL PRODUCTS

Binoculars
Monocular

- Many people continue to play golf with low vision. Align the ball, your shoulders, and the club carefully before you swing and let your experience carry your stroke. Use your binoculars or monocular to see the putting green. Ask a friend to stand by the hole for better visibility during putting.

- Bowling is another game you can play with low vision. Aim for the black lane markers near your feet and consider using a lighter ball for easier aim. Use your binoculars or monocular to see which pins are still standing or ask a teammate.

- Consider taking gentle yoga, stretching, or tai chi classes. Tell the instructor that you have low vision and stand or sit up front. Many instructors teach these classes by orally explaining all the moves, so your low vision will not interrupt the class and you will be able to follow the instructor.

- Consider joining a local senior-friendly health club. Many clubs cater to a young clientele, but others have senior members. Clubs may provide staff-assisted weight-training programs, stationary bicycles, rowing machines, and lap swimming pools. If you do not swim, you can purchase an inexpensive pool running belt that holds you upright and afloat while you run in the water. Athletes use pool running as a gentle, effective training routine when they are recovering from knee and ankle injuries because it provides good aerobic exercise that's easy on your joints. Alternatively, use a kickboard to kick across the pool or join a water-aerobics class.

- Walk for exercise. Attach a lightweight pair of binoculars or monocular to a cord around your neck for easy street sign reading and street crossings. You can also walk with a friend. Take your friend's upper arm and let them walk freely while you use his or her arm for guidance as needed. Do not let someone take your arm and guide you, since they may unwittingly throw you off balance.

AIRPLANES AND TRAVELING

- If your gate is far away request assistance when you check in.

- You can also request a seat close to the screen. You can use the same glasses for in-flight movies that you use for watching television at home.

- Use your lighted hand-held magnifier for reading tickets, and your binoculars or monocular for seeing gate numbers.

- Put brightly colored, contrasting tape on both sides of your luggage so it will be more

---

SELECTED HELPFUL PRODUCTS

Light-yellow sunglasses for glare
Portable tape player and books on
    tape
Lighted hand-held magnifier
Binoculars, monocular, TV glasses

Portable magnifying mirror
Portable large-print alarm clock
Large-print telephone and address
    books
Brightly colored or large-print luggage
    tags

---

easily identifiable. Purchase or make yourself big-print luggage tags with black block lettering.

- Wear your low vision button or carry your white identification cane, and tell the airline staff that you have low vision. Low vision entitles you to preboard the plane, giving you more time to find your seat and arrange your belongings before other passengers crowd the aisles and jostle for overhead luggage space. Preboarding is no small advantage during holiday travel times and will save you much stress.

- Make sure that the flight attendant serving you knows that you have low vision. He or she will make a special effort to hand you drinks so that you can see them, or help open those hard-to-see foil tops on airline juice containers.

RETURNING HOME

Keys and Keyholes

- Keys often look alike. Label your look-alike keys with stick-on felt tabs or safety pins. Put the key you use most on the outside of the ring. You can also put keys on separate brightly colored plastic key rings.
- Use your flashlight to see keyholes in greater

detail. To help aim your key, put a finger on the keyhole and aim the key toward that finger.

Alarms

- If the buttons on your home alarm are the same color as the alarm or the wall, mark them with bright stickers or puff paint (see the supplies list in Chapter 9). Sometimes it can be difficult to remember an alarm combination or the alarm keypad configuration if you can't see the numbers on the buttons. To help jog your memory, try making a map. Draw a big picture of the alarm keypad using a thick black marker on a white 8.5-by-11-inch piece of paper. Put the paper on the wall next to the alarm.

Mailboxes and Packages

- If your mailbox is one of many in a bank of boxes, mark it with contrasting tape or stickers. If someone removes the tape, inform the building manager that you have low vision and you need to distinguish your mailbox from the rest in order to see it clearly.

- If your walk is icy or you have trouble balancing, always carry fewer items and make more trips rather than trying to carry everything at once. Unpack bags and packages and put things away when you return so that piles don't accumulate, making it difficult to see other items.

Welcome Home

- When you return home, put your keys in their regular place so that they'll be ready next time. And give yourself credit for having gone out and done whatever you needed or wanted to do in the world.

Congratulations on finishing this rehabilitation program! Sometimes visual rehabilitation can feel overwhelming, especially if you've only recently lost vision, or if you are experiencing depression. But keep going! Reach out to the resources that you have in this book, in the appendices, in your communities, with your family and friends, and within yourself. Keep your heart and your humor. We're rooting for you. You can do it.

PART IV

Appendices

APPENDIX I

National Organizations, Books, and Audiotapes

TO FIND A VISUAL REHABILITATION PROGRAM IN YOUR AREA, CONTACT THE FOLLOWING ORGANIZATIONS:

American Foundation for the Blind (AFB)
11 Penn Plaza, Suite 300
New York, NY 10001
212-502-7600
Fax: 212-502-7777
E-Mail: newyork@afb.org
www.afb.org
Provides information on resources, publishes materials and a newsletter. Developer of books on tape. Career and Technology Information Bank: 212-502-7642.

REGIONAL OFFICES OF AFB

AFB Midwest
401 N. Michigan Avenue, Suite 308
Chicago, IL 60611
312-245-9961
Fax: 312-245-9965
E-mail: chicago@afb.org

AFB West
111 Pine Street, Suite 725
San Francisco, CA 94111
415-392-4845
Fax: 415-392-0383
E-mail: sanfran@afb.org

AFB Southwest
260 Treadway Plaza, Exchange Park
Dallas, TX 75235
214-352-7222
Fax: 214-352-3214
E-mail: afbdallas@afb.org

AFB Southeast
100 Peachtree Street, Suite 620
Atlanta, GA 30303
404-525-2303
Fax: 404-659-6957
E-mail: atlanta@afb.org

Foundation Fighting Blindness

1401 Mt. Royal Ave., 4th Floor
Baltimore, MD 21217
800-683-5551

Many local chapters, meetings, support groups; funds research, provides updated information

The Lighthouse, Inc.

111 East 59th Street
New York, NY 10022
212-821-9200
800-334-5497
www.lighthouse.org
Information and Resource Caller Service
800-829-0500

Provides information on visual rehabilitation services nationwide, instruction courses for professionals, research on effects of vision loss and advocacy. Also direct visual rehabilitation services and retail shop serving metropolitan New York, as well as catalog of books, optical and non-optical devices.

National Association for the Visually Handicapped (NAVH)

22 West 21st Street
New York, NY 10010
212-889-3141
800-677-9965
Fax: 212-727-2931
E-mail: staff@navh.org
www.navh.org
(continued)

and

3201 Balboa Street
San Francisco, CA 94121
415-221-3201
Fax: 415-221-8754
E-mail: staffca@navh.org

Provides information regarding visual rehabilitation programs nationwide, publishes worldwide quarterly newsletter and educational materials
about vision in English, Russian, and Spanish, offers
free large-print loan library nationwide and visual
aids by catalog and Web site. Sale and training in
use of equipment at both sites. Nonprofit, chari-
table, membership organization.

U.S. Dept. of Veterans Affairs
Blind Rehab Service
531 TECH
810 Vermont Ave NW
Washington, DC 20420
202-535-7637

Extensive visual rehabilitation for veterans at
regional inpatient centers. Visual aids provided.

PROFESSIONAL ORGANIZATIONS

American Academy of Ophthalmology
Low Vision Committee
655 Beach Street
San Francisco, CA 94109-1336
415-561-8500

American Academy of Optometry
6110 Executive Blvd.
Rockville, MD 20852
301-984-1441

American Occupational Therapy Association
4720 Montgomery Lane, P.O. Box 31220
Bethesda, MD 20824-1220
301-652-AOTA
800-377-8555

American Optometric Association
Low Vision Section
243 North Lindbergh Blvd.
St. Louis, MO 63141
314-991-4100

Association for the Education and Rehabilitation of the Blind and Visually Impaired
P.O. Box 22387
Alexandria, VA 22304
703-823-9690
www.aerbvi.org

MACULAR DEGENERATION ORGANIZATIONS

The Association for Macular Diseases
210 East 64th Street
New York, NY 10021
212-605-3719
Large-print newsletter, information, resources; subscription by membership; nonprofit.

Macular Degeneration International
2968 W. Ina Road, #106
Tucson, AZ 85741
520-797-2525
Large-print newsletter, information, resources; subscription by membership; nonprofit.

Macular Degeneration Foundation
P.O. Box 9752
San Jose, CA 95157
408-260-1335
888-633-3937
www.eyesight.org
e-mail: eyesight@eyesight.org
Develops and supports research on ARMD. Quarterly free newsletter with research updates.

LOW VISION READING WORKBOOKS

Learn to Use Your Vision for Reading
(LUV Reading) Workbook
Mattingly International
938-K Andreasen Drive
Escondido, CA 92024
800-826-4200

McGill Low Vision Manual
Betacom Group
2999 King Street
W. Inglewood, Ont. LON1KO Canada
800-353-1107

LARGE PRINT BOOKS

Doubleday Large Print Home Library
6550 East 30th Street
Indianapolis, IN 46206-6325
800-688-4442
    Book club for large-print books: specified number to be purchased at regular price and additional special offers.

ISIS Large Print Books
Transaction Publishers
Rutgers-The State U. of New Jersey
New Brunswick, NJ 08903
732-445-2280

Catalog of large-print books for purchase. Over 250 American and British titles.

Jewish Heritage for the Blind
1655 E. 24th Street
Brooklyn, NY 11229
718-338-4999
Free large-print religious readings; requires statement from doctor confirming low vision.

The Large Print Literary Reader
958 Massachusetts Ave. #105
Cambridge, MA 02139
800-216-5893
Only literary magazine in large print; monthly issues, by subscription.

National Association for Visually Handicapped (NAVH)
See under "Organizations"
Free lending library of large-print books.

The New York Times Large Type Weekly
P.O. Box 9564
Uniondale, NY 11555-9564
800-631-2580
Selected articles, large (2M) print, approx. 36 pages.

Random House Large Type Division
400 Hahn Road
Westminster, MD 21157
800-733-3000
　　Distributor of large-print books. Will send list of available titles upon request. May order through them, with shipping charge, or through bookstore.

Reader's Digest Large Edition
P.O. Box 751
Mount Morris, IL 61054-8442
800-678-9746
　　Same content as regular edition, large (2M) print.

AUDIOTAPES (SELECTED LIST)

American Printing House for The Blind
1839 Frankfort Avenue
P.O. Box 6085
Louisville, KY 40206-0085
800-223-1839
Fax: 502-895-1509
　　Provides *Newsweek* and *Reader's Digest* free on cassette tape. Ask about their large-print books, too. They have a very large collection.

Choice Magazine Listening
85 Channel Drive
Port Washington, NY 10050
516-883-8280

Selected readings, free for those registered with Library of Congress Talking Book Program.

National Library Service for the Blind
Library of Congress Talking Book Program
1291 Taylor Street, NW
Washington, DC 20542
202-707-5100
800-424-8567

Vast selection of books on tape, free, as a national service. Register through your county library, which supplies tape player. Semimonthly catalogs and easy, free mailing system. Requires statement from physician of physical or visual impairment causing inability to read standard print.

Radio Reading Services
To find in your area, call Commission for the Blind or local radio stations.

Local radio stations use volunteers to read local and national publications for broadcast on special frequency to receivers supplied to visually impaired listeners.

The Bible Alliance
P.O. Box 621
Bradenton, FL 34206
941-748-3031
Fax: 941-748-2625

Free Bible on audiocassette. New Testament in fifty-two languages. Selected books of Old Testament in English, German, Hebrew, Italian, Luganda, and Spanish. Requires physician's statement of visual impairment.

Product Catalogs, Retailers, Computers, and Software

LOW VISION PRODUCT CATALOGS (SELECTED LIST)

Independent Living Aids, Inc.
27 East Mall
Plainview, NY 11803
800-537-2118
Fax: 516-752-3135
    Medium-size print catalog with color pictures. Magnifiers and non-optical aids and NOIR glasses.

LS&S Group, Inc.
P.O. Box 673
Northbrook, IL 60065
800-468-4789
Fax: 847-498-1482
E-mail: LSSGRP@aol.com
    Small-size print catalog, black-and-white pictures. Best catalog for magnifiers, very wide selection, but also more complicated to read. Offers non-optical aids and NOIR glasses.

The Lighthouse, Inc.
Consumer Products Division
36-20 Northern Boulevard
Long Island City, NY 11101
800-829-0500

    Large-print catalog with color pictures. Easy to read, offers magnifiers and non-optical aids. Also offers good ideas for holiday gifts.

Nat'l Assoc. for Visually Handicapped
22 West 21st Street, 6th Floor
New York, NY 10010
212-737-2931
E-mail: staff@navh.org
www.navh.org

    Catalog free to members, $2.50 for nonmembers. Large print with big black-and-white pictures, easy to read, also includes resource references.

NOIR Medical Technologies
P.O. Box 159
6155 Pontiac Trail
South Lyon, MI 48178
800-521-9746
Fax: 734-769-1708

    Small-print catalog, targeted to doctors; offers NOIR tinted glasses, many shades and styles.

CCTV MANUFACTURERS AND RETAILERS (SELECTED LIST)

Enhanced Vision Systems
2130 Main Street, Ste 250
Huntington Beach, CA 92648
800-440-9476
Fax 714-374-1821
www.enchancedvision.com
"Max" hand-held camera-mouse plugs into your TV. Provides 30X magnification on 20-inch television screen.

Innoventions, Inc.
5921 S. Middlefield Road, Suite 102
Littleton, CO 80123-2877
800-854-6554
Fax: 303-727-4940
E-mail: magnicam@magnicam.com
www.magnicam.com/magnicam
"Magni-Cam" hand-held camera plugs into your TV; 4X to 70X variable with screen size. Color model, head-mounted unit and portable screen available also.

Magnisight, Inc.
P.O. Box 2653
Colorado Springs, CO 80901
800-753-4767
Camera and screen units separate, can be stacked or side-by-side, camera available sepa-

rately; to 45X with 4-inch screen, to 60X with 19-inch. Portable model 18X with 7-inch screen.

Optelec
6 Lyberty Way, P.O. Box 729
Westford, MA 01886
800-828-1056

Several camera-screen units, including "20/20": 3X to 60X, 14-inch screen; "20/20+": 20- inch screen, choice of color, computer connection; "20/20 Spectrum": 5X to 60X full color. Also see under Computers.

TeleSensory, Inc.
455 N. Bernardo Ave.
Mountain View, CA 94043-5237
800-804-8004
Fax: 415-335-1816

Several models of camera-screen units: "Aladdin" 14-inch screen; "Aladdin Rainbow" with 6 color choices; "Aladdin Genie," color, computer connection.

HEAD-MOUNTED VIEWING DEVICES

Enhanced Vision Systems
800-440-9476
(see above under CCTV)

"V-Max" 23 ounce head-mounted color camera and display system, focusable for far and near. Also plugs into your TV, to become 60X CCTV.

LOW VISION COMPUTERS AND SOFTWARE (SELECTED LIST)

Arkenstone
1390 Borregas Avenue
Sunnyvale, CA 94089
800-444-4443
Fax: 408-745-6739
E-mail: info@arkenstone.org
 IBM-compatible software with voice synthesizer computers: Optical Character Recognition (OCR) systems, personal reading machines.

Artic Technologies
55 Park St., Suite 2
Troy, MI 48083-2753
810-588-7370
Fax: 810-588-2650
 Software to enlarge computer text, make Windows accessible; voice synthesizers for computers.

Berkeley Systems
2095 Rose St.
Berkeley, CA 94709
510-540-5535
 "InLarge" software to enlarge Macintosh computer text.

HumanWare, Inc.
6245 King Road
Loomis, CA 95650
800-722-3393
Fax: 916-652-7296

Large-print computer software, voice synthesizers.

IBM Independence Series
P.O. Box 1328
Boca Raton, FL 33429-1328
800-426-4832

Software to make Windows accessible; voice synthesizers for computers.

TeleSensory, Inc.
455 N. Bernardo Ave.
P.O. Box 7455
Mountainview, CA 94039-7455
800-227-8418

"Vista" software to enlarge computer text and "ScreenPower" voice synthesizer program. (See also under CCTVs.)

Xerox Imaging Systems
9 Centennial Park Drive
Peabody, MA 01960
800-421-7323

Voice synthesizers for computers and personal reading machines (OCRs). (See also under CCTVs.)

Transportation Information, Driving Regulations, and Taxes

TRANSPORTATION INFORMATION

Public Transportation
Local Mass Transit Authority or
State Office on Aging or Disability
Transportation service provided by many communities at low cost for senior citizens and those with visual and other physical impairments.

Volunteer Transportation
Call local Office on Aging, Senior Center, Elks, Lions Club, Knights of Columbus, or your church.

Private Transportation
Allot funds otherwise used for car payments, insurance, and fuel to taxi fares or hired driver wages.

Alternative Transportation (1)
Three-wheeled bicycle, with basket for shopping.

Alternative Transportation (2)

Battery operated three or four wheel sidewalk vehicles. Travel at walking speed, safe for most "drivers" with ARMD. Go through doorways, can have baskets, use inside and outside. Some larger two-seaters. Recommend bicycle flag for visibility to auto drivers since rider crosses streets at chair height.

SOURCES OF BATTERY OPERATED VEHICLES:

Amigo Mobility International, Inc.
6693 Dixie Highway
Bridgeport, MI 48722
517-777-0910

Electric Mobility
1 Mobility Plaza
Sewell, NJ 08080
800-662-4548

Lark of America
P.O. Box 1647
Waukesha, WI 53187-1647
800-537-1600

Palmer Industries
P.O. Box 5707HG
Endicott, NY 13763
800-847-1304
www.palmerind.com

Sears Shop-at-Home
Sears Tower
Chicago, IL 60684
800-326-1750

VISUAL REQUIREMENTS FOR DRIVING

Most states require 20/40 vision in one eye for an unrestricted driver's license, although some allow residents with lower vision to drive. The visual requirements for a restricted license vary from 20/60 to 20/200. Some states allow selected drivers to use specially fitted telescopes with appropriate training and road testing or issue restricted licences that allow driving only on local streets or during the day. Call your Secretary of State's office to find out the laws in your state.

TAX BENEFITS

If you qualify as legally blind and you do not itemize, you are eligible for a $700 federal tax exemption. Legal blindness means that your best corrected vision is not better than 20/200 in either eye, and that your visual field is 20 degrees or less. See your optometrist or ophthalmologist for visual testing and documentation of legal blindness.

APPENDIX IV

Selected Bibliography

Beaver Dam Eye Study:

Klein, Ronald, M.D., Barbara E. K. Klein, M.D., Susan C. Jensen, M.S. "The Relation of Cardiovascular Disease and Its Risk Factors to the 5-Year Incidence of Age-Related Maculopathy: The Beaver Dam Eye Study." *Ophthalmology,* 104:11, 1804–1812, November 1997.

Klein, Ronald, M.D., Barbara E. K. Klein, M.D., Susan C. Jensen, M.S., Stacy M. Meuer, B.S. "The Five-Year Incidence and Progression of Age-Related Maculopathy: The Beaver Dam Eye Study." *Ophthalmology,* 104:1, 7–21, January 1997.

Klein, Ronald, M.D., Barbara E. K. Klein, M.D., M.P.H., Scott E. Moss, M.A. "Diabetes, Hyperglycemia, and Age-Related Maculopathy: The Beaver Dam Eye Study." *Ophthalmology,* 99:10, 1527–1533, October 1992.

Klein, Ronald, M.D., M.P.H., Barbara E. K. Klein, M.D., M.P.H., and Kathryn L. P.

Linton, M.S. "Prevalence of Age-Related Maculopathy: The Beaver Dam Eye Study." *Ophthalmology,* 99:6, 933–943, June 1992.

Bressler, Neil M., M.D., and Susan B. Bressler, M.D. "Preventive Ophthalmology: Age-Related Macular Degeneration." *Ophthalmology,* 102:8, 1206–1211, August 1995.

Bressler, Susan B., M.D. "Age-Related Macular Degeneration." *Focal Points,* The American Academy of Ophthalmology, 8:2, 1–14, March 1995.

Carlsen, Mary Baird, Ph.D. *Creative Aging: A Meaning-Making Perspective.* New York: Norton, 1991.

Cole, Roy G., O.D., F.A.A.O., and Bruce P. Rosenthal, O.D., F.A.A.O. *Remediation and Management of Low Vision.* New York: Mosby, 1996.

Cole, Thomas R. *The Journey of Life: A Cultural History of Aging in America.* Cambridge: Cambridge University Press, 1992.

Colenbrander, August, M.D., and Donald C. Fletcher, M.D., guest eds. *Ophthalmology Clinics of North America.* Philadelphia: W. B. Saunders Company, June 1994.

Cruickshanks, Karen J., Ph.D., et al. "The Prevalence of Age-Related Maculopathy by Geographic Region and Ethnicity." *Archives of Ophthalmology,* 115, 242–250, February 1997.

Darzins, Peteris, B.M., B.S., Paul Mitchell, M.D.,

Richard R. Heller, M.D. "Sun Exposure and Age-Related Macular Degeneration: An Australian Case-Control Study." *Ophthalmology,* 104:5, 770–776, May 1997.

Delany, Sarah and A. Elizabeth Delany. *Having Our Say.* New York: Kodansha, 1993.

Dickinson, Annette, Ph.D., ed. *Benefits of Nutritional Supplements.* Washington, DC: Council for Responsible Nutrition, 1993.

Erikson, Erik H., Joan M. Erikson, and Helen Q. Kivnick. *Vital Involvement in Old Age.* New York: Norton, 1986.

Eye Disease Case-Control Study Group. "Antioxidant Status and Neovascular Age-Related Macular Degeneration." *Archives of Ophthalmology,* 111, 104–109, January 1993.

Faye, Eleanor E., M.D. "Guide to Selecting Reading Spectacles, Hand Magnifiers, Stand Magnifiers, Telescopes, Electronic Aids, and Absorptive Lenses." In *Clinical Low Vision*, 2d ed., Eleanor E. Faye, M.D., ed. Boston: Little, Brown and Company, 1984.

Friedman, Ephraim, M.D. "The Pathogenesis of Age-Related Macular Degeneration and Its Potential Prevention." *Research to Prevent Blindness Eye Research Seminar,* 44–46, October 1995.

Goldberg, Jack, Gordon Flowerdew, Ellen Smith, Jacob A. Brody, and Mark Tso, O.M. "Factors

Associated with Age-Related Macular Degeneration." *American Journal of Epidemiology,* 128:4, 700–710.

Goldman, Connie and Richard Mahler. *Secrets of Becoming a Late Bloomer: Extraordinary Ordinary People on the Art of Staying Creative, Alive, and Aware in Mid-Life and Beyond.* Walpole, NH: Stillpoint Press, 1995.

Goleman, Daniel. *Emotional Intelligence.* New York: Bantam, 1995.

Hamer, Dean, Ph.D., and Peter Copeland. *Living with Our Genes: Why They Matter More Than You Think.* New York: Doubleday, 1998.

Hampton, G. Robert, and Philip T. Nelson, eds. *Age-Related Macular Degeneration: Principles and Practice.* New York: Raven Press, Ltd., 1992.

Heilbrun, Carolyn G. *The Last Gift of Time: Life Beyond Sixty.* New York: Ballantine, 1997.

Hemingway, Ernest. *The Old Man and the Sea.* New York: Simon & Schuster, 1952.

Hirvela, Heli, M.D., Heikki Luukinen, M.D., Esa Laard, Lic. Sc., Leila Laatikainen, M.D. "Risk Factors of Age-Related Maculopathy in a Population 70 Years of Age or Older." *Ophthalmology,* 103:6, 871–877, June 1996.

Ivers, Rebecca Q., M.P.H., Robert G. Cumming, M.B., B.S., M.P.H., Ph.D., Paul Mitchell, M.D., and Karin Attebo, M.B., B.S. "Visual Impairment and Falls in Older Adults: The Blue Mountains Eye Study." *Journal of the American Geriatrics Society,* 46, 58–64, 1998.

Jose, Randall, ed. *Understanding Low Vision.* New York: American Foundation for the Blind, 1983.

Kabat-Zinn, Jon, Ph.D. *Wherever You Go There You Are.* New York: Hyperion, 1994.

———. *Full Catastrophe Living: Using the Wisdom of Your Body and Mind to Face Stress, Pain, and Illness.* New York: Delta, 1990.

Lee, Paul P., M.D., J.D., Karen Spritzer, M.A., Ron D. Hays, Ph.D. "The Impact of Blurred Vision on Functioning and Well-Being." *Ophthalmology,* 104:3, 390–396, March 1997.

Macular Photocoagulation Study (individual authors not listed in original studies):

Macular Photocoagulation Study Group. "Risk Factors for Choroidal Neovascularization in the Second Eye of Patients with Juxtafoveal or Subfoveal Choroidal Neovascularization Secondary to Age-Related Macular Degeneration." *Archives of Ophthalmology,* 115, 741–747, June 1997.

Macular Photocoagulation Study Group. "Laser Photocoagulation of Subfoveal Neovascular Lesions of Age-Related Macular Degeneration." *Archives of Ophthalmology,* 111, 1200–1209, September 1993.

Macular Photocoagulation Study Group. "Five-Year Follow-Up of Fellow Eyes of Patients with Age-Related Macular Degeneration and Unilateral Extrafoveal Choroidal Neovascularization." *Archives of Ophthalmology,* 111, 1189–1199, September 1993.

Macular Photocoagulation Study Group. "Recurrent Choroidal Neovascularization After Argon Laser Photocoagulation for Neovascular Maculopathy." *Archives of Ophthalmology,* 104, 503–513, April 1986.

Macular Photocoagulation Study Group. "Argon Laser Photocoagulation for Neovascular Maculopathy: Five Year Results from Randomized Clinical Trials." *Archives of Ophthalmology,* 109, 1109–1114, August 1991.

Mangels, Ann Reed, Ph.D., Joanne M. Holden, M.S., Gary R. Beecher, Ph.D., Michele R. Forman, Ph.D., Elaine Lanza, Ph.D. "Carotenoid Content of Fruits and Vegetables: An Evaluation of Analytic Data." *Journal of the American Dietetic Association,* 93:3, 284–296, March 1993.

Mares-Perlman, Julie A., Ph.D., et al. "Association of Zinc and Antioxidant Nutrients With Age-Related Maculopathy." *Archives of Ophthalmology,* 114, 991–997, August 1996.

Mares-Perlman, Julie A., Ph.D. "Diet and Ocular Disease." *Research to Prevent Blindness Eye Research Seminar,* 42–44, October 1995.

Selected Bibliography

Miller, Merle. *Plain Speaking: An Oral Biography of Harry S. Truman.* New York: Berkley, 1973.

Mitchell, Paul, M.D. FRACO, Wayne Smith, B.Med., M.P.H, Jai Jin Wang, NMED. "Iris Color, Skin Sensitivity and Age Related Maculopathy: The Blue Mountain Eye Study," *Ophthalmology,* 105, 1359–63, August 1998.

Murray, Michael T., N.D. *Encyclopedia of Nutritional Supplements.* Rocklin, CA: Prima Publishing, 1996.

Newsome, David A., M.D., Mano Swartz, M.D., Nicholas C. Leone, M.D., Robert C. Elston, Ph.D., Earl Miller. "Oral Zinc in Macular Degeneration." *Archives of Ophthalmology,* 106, 192–198, February 1988.

Norden, Michael J., M.D. *Beyond Prozac: Brain Toxic Lifestyles, Natural Antidotes & New Generation Antidepressants.* New York: Harper-Collins, 1995.

Nowakowski, Rodney W. *Primary Low Vision Care.* Norwalk, CT: Appleton and Lange, 1994.

Podmore, Ian D., et al. "Vitamin C Exhibits Pro-Oxidant Properties." *Nature* 392, April 9, 1998.

Pollack, Ayala, M.D., Arie Marcovitch, M.D., Amir Bukelman, M.D., Moshe Oliver, M.D. "Age-Related Macular Degeneration after Extracapsular Cataract Extraction with Intra-ocular Lens Implantation." *Ophthalmology,* 103:10, 1546–1554, October 1996.

Preziosi, Paul, M.D., et al. "Effects of Supplementation with a Combination of Antioxidant Vitamins and Trace Elements, at Nutritional Doses, on Biochemical Indicators and Markers of the Antioxidant System in Adult Subjects." *Journal of the American College of Nutrition,* 17:5, 244–249, June 1998.

Reinhardt, Joann P. "The Importance of Friendship and Family Support in Adaptation to Chronic Vision Impairment." *Journal of Gerontology,* 51B:5, 268–278, 1996.

Rodale Press. *Healing with Vitamins.* Emmaus, PA: Rodale Press, 1996.

Rosenthal, Bruce P., O.D., F.A.A.O., and Roy G. Cole, O.D., F.A.A.O. *Functional Assessment of Low Vision.* New York: Mosby-Year Book, Inc., 1996.

Ross, Robert D., et al. "Presumed Macular Choroidal Watershed Vascular Filling, Choroidal Neovascularization, and Systemic Vascular Disease in Patients With Age-Related Macular Degeneration." *American Journal of Ophthalmology,* 125:1 71–80, January 1998.

Rowe, John W., M.D., and Robert L. Kahn, Ph.D. *Successful Aging: The MacArthur Foundation Study.* New York: Pantheon, 1998.

Saint Exupéry, Antoine de. *The Little Prince.* New York: Harcourt, Brace & World, Inc., 1943.

Schachter-Shalomi, Zalman, and Ronald S.

Miller. *From Ageing to Sage-ing: A Profound New Vision of Growing Older.* New York: Warner Books, 1995.

Seddon, Johanna M., M.D., and the Eye Disease Case-Control Study Group. "Dietary Carotenoids, Vitamins A, C, and E, and Advanced Age-Related Macular Degeneration." *Journal of the AMA (JAMA)*, 272:8, 1413–1420, November 9, 1994.

Siegel, Bernie, M.D. "Healing From the Inside Out." Carlsbad, CA: Hays House, 1997.

Smith, Wayne, M.P.H., Paul Mitchell, M.D., Stephen R. Leeder, Ph.D. "Smoking and Age-Related Maculopathy: The Blue Mountains Eye Study." *Archives of Ophthalmology*, 114, 1518–1523, December 1996.

Snodderly, D. Max, Ph.D. "Evidence for Protection Against Age-Related Macular Degeneration by Carotenoids and Antioxidant Vitamins." *American Journal of Clinical Nutrition*, 62 (supplement), 1448S–61S, 1995.

Spaide, Richard F., et al. "External Beam Radiation Therapy for Choroidal Neovascularization." *Ophthalmology*, 105:1, 24–30, January 1998.

Weil, Andrew, M.D. *Natural Health, Natural Medicine.* New York: Houghton Mifflin, 1998.

———. *Eight Weeks to Optimum Health.* New York: Knopf, 1997.

Werbach, Melvyn, R., M.D. *Nutritional Influences on Illness.* Tarzana, CA: Third Line Press, 1996.

West, Sheila K., Ph.D., et al. "Exposure to Sunlight and Other Risk Factors for Age-Related Macular Degeneration." *Archives of Ophthalmology,* 107, 875–879, June 1989.

West, Sheila, Ph.D., et al. "Are Antioxidants or Supplements Protective for Age-Related Macular Degeneration?" *Archives of Ophthalmology,* 112, 222–227, February 1994.

Williams, Rebecca A., Ph.D., Barbara L. Brody, M.P.H., Ronald G. Thomas, Ph.D., Robert M. Kaplan, Ph.D., Stuart I. Brown, M.D. "The Psychosocial Impact of Macular Degeneration." *Socioeconomics of Ophthalmology, The Archives of Ophthalmology* 116, 514–520, April 1998.

Young, Richard W., Ph.D. "Solar Radiation and Age-Related Macular Degeneration." *Survey of Ophthalmology,* 32:4, 252–269, January–February 1988.

Young, Richard W., Ph.D. "Pathophysiology of Age-Related Macular Degeneration." *Survey of Ophthalmology,* 31:5, 291–306, March–April 1987.

Zeuss, Jonathan, M.D. *The Natural Prozac Program: How to Use St. John's Wort, the Antidepressant Herb.* New York: Three Rivers Press, 1997.

BOOKS AND ARTICLES BY PEOPLE WITH MACULAR DEGENERATION

Grunwald, Henry. "Losing Sight." In *The New Yorker*, December 9, 1996, 62–67.

Neer, Frances. *Dancing in The Dark*. Berkeley, CA: Creative Arts Publishing, 1994.

Ringgold, Nicolette Pernot. *Out of the Corner of My Eye: Living With Vision Loss in Later Life*. New York: American Foundation for the Blind, 1991.

See, Carolyn. "Going Blind and Fighting In Every Possible Way." *Modern Maturity*. September–October 1997, 47–49.

Silverman, Bert. *Bert's Eye View: Coping with Macular Degeneration*. Portland, ME.: Viewpoint Press, 1997.

About the Authors

LYLAS G. MOGK, M.D., is a practicing ophthalmologist and founding Director of the Visual Rehabilitation and Research Center of Michigan, part of the Henry Ford Health System. Dr. Mogk is a member of the American Academy of Ophthalmology's Low Vision Rehabilitation Committee. She lives in Grosse Pointe with her husband, John, and her father, Charles R. Good, who has advanced macular degeneration. Despite his severe vision loss, Dr. Mogk's father lives a full and active life following the principles presented in this book.

MARJA MOGK is a freelance writer and editor based in Berkeley, California. She worked for several years in social welfare counseling and maintains an active interest in this field. She is Lylas and John Mogk's daughter.